Study Guide for

Rambo's Nursing Skills for Clinical Practice

Fourth Edition

Susan C. deWit, MSN, RNCS

Instructor of Nursing
El Centro College
Dallas, Texas

W.B. SAUNDERS COMPANY
A Division of Harcourt Brace & Company
Philadelphia London Toronto Montreal Sydney Tokyo

W. B. Saunders Company
A Division of
Harcourt Brace & Company

The Curtis Center
Independence Square West
Philadelphia, PA 19106

Study Guide for
RAMBO'S NURSING SKILLS
FOR CLINICAL PRACTICE
Fourth Edition

Copyright © 1994 by W.B. Saunders Company
All rights reserved.No part of this publication may be reproduced or transmitted in any form or by any means, electronic or mechanical, including photocopy, recording, or any information storage and retrieval system, without permission in writing from the publisher.

Permission is hereby granted to reproduce the Performance Checklists in this publication in complete pages, with the copyright notice, for instructional use and not for resale.

Printed in the United States of America

ISBN 0-7216-4324-8

Last digit is the print number: 9   8   7   6   5   4   3

Contents

Preface

This *Study Guide* is designed to reinforce and enhance learning of the material in the accompanying *Rambo's Nursing Skills for Clinical Practice, 4th Ed*. The study guide consists of study questions for each chapter, performance checklists for each skill covered in the text, and suggestions for activities that will broaden learning and experience in the clinical area.

It is suggested that the student first read the text chapter, noting the chapter objectives, then complete the study questions. The post-test should be taken as the last exercise. The answers to the study questions are located in the *Instructor's Manual;* the answers to the post-test for each chapter in the text are located at the back of the text. The Introduction in the text entitled "Student Survival Skills" should assist the student to study efficiently.

Reading through the suggested clinical activities before the clinical experience will help the student plan on ways to apply new skills in the clinical setting and focus on various means of broadening knowledge and experience. The more a skill can be practiced at home or in the skill laboratory, the more confidence the student will have when doing it in the clinical setting.

Each school's instructors will notify students if there are any "critical elements" among the steps of each performance checklist. A "critical element" is a step that must be performed with 100% accuracy in order for the skill performance to be acceptable for a "pass" designation. "Critical elements" should be marked before students begin practicing the skill. The Standard Steps of identifying the patient, checking orders, explaining the procedure, providing privacy, and promoting safety are considered "critical elements" in most schools.

A good way to practice a skill is to first slowly go through it by reading a step, performing the step, verifying correct performance, and then progressing to the next step. When this stage is completed, the student should ask a peer to watch, and then go through the entire skill procedure, only verifying sequence of steps or correct way to perform a step as needed. When confident that the skill is mastered, the student should have the peer partner evaluate the skill performance as it is completed. If performance is satisfactory, the student is ready for instructor evaluation and then skill performance in the clinical setting.

The author welcomes comments and suggestions on the text and supplemental materials. Send comments to:

Susan deWit, MSN, RNCS
c/o Thomas Eoyang
Editor-in-Chief
W.B. Saunders Company
The Curtis Center
Independence Square West
Philadelphia, PA 19106-3399

Standard Steps for Nursing Procedures

The following steps are followed at the beginning of each nursing procedure:

IMPORTANT STEPS	KEY POINTS/RATIONALE
A. Check the order, collect the equipment and supplies, and wash hands. • Verify the order • Check the agency's policy and procedure manual for accepted method of performing this procedure	Not all procedures require an order. The correct equipment and supplies are necessary to perform the procedure.
• Process equipment and supply charges • Wash your hands	Supplies and equipment use must be charged to the patient. Washing hands prevents taking organisms from the chart, nurse's station and supply room to the patient.
B. Identify and prepare the patient. • Greet the patient and introduce yourself • Check the patient's identification band • Explain what you are going to do • Answer any questions	Preparation for a procedure places the patient more at ease. Identifying the patient correctly according to agency policy each and every time a procedure is performed prevents errors. Explaining the procedure reduces fear of the unknown. Using terms the patient can understand for your explanation establishes rapport and aids comprehension
C. Provide privacy and institute safety precautions; arrange the supplies and equipment.	The patient has a right to privacy.

IMPORTANT STEPS	KEY POINTS/RATIONALE
• Close the door or curtains and drape the patient as needed • Avoid a loud voice when discussing what is to be done	
• Raise the bed to working height; be certain the bed is in locked position; raise siderails before turning or leaving the patient	Raising the bed to working height, being certain the bed is in locked position, and raising siderails before turning or leaving the patient prevents falls and protects the patient's safety.
• Check equipment for breaks, wear, and safety	For safety, equipment must be in good working order.
• Set up the equipment and supplies in an orderly, methodical fashion for use	Efficiency requires setting up equipment and supplies in the order in which things will be used.
D. Use Universal precautions and aseptic technique as appropriate.	Universal precautions are to be used with every patient.
• Wear gloves when there is a possibility of coming in contact with blood or other body fluids	Gloves act as a barrier between the contaminant and the skin.
• Wear protective eyewear and an impermeable gown or apron when there is any danger of being splashed with blood or body fluids	Protective eyewear and an impermeable gown act as barriers.

Important Steps	Key Points/Rationale	Important Steps	Key Points/Rationale
D. (continued)		X. (continued)	
• Use sharp instruments and needles carefully and follow protocols to prevent injury	Attentive, careful use with sharp objects, helps prevent injuries.	• To remove gloves without contaminating yourself, begin by pulling one glove off without touching your skin; hold the glove removed in the palm of the remaining gloved hand and then reach to the inside of the other glove and roll it down the hand. Dispose of the gloves in the trash	
• Do not recap needles without a needle recapping device	Universal precaution guidelines state that needles should not be recapped		
• Dispose of all sharps by dropping them into a sharps container. See Appendix III in text for specifics of Universal Precautions	Sharps are to be dropped into a sharps container for disposal.		
		• Wash your hands immediately	Universal precautions requires handwashing immediately after removing gloves
E. Perform the task according to protocol:	For legal protection, procedures must be performed according to agency policies and protocols.	Y. Resore the unit:	
• Mentally review the steps of the task beforehand		a. Make the person comfortable.	Safety and order must be restored for patient well-being.
• If you are uncertain how to do a task, ask your team leader, resource nurse, instructor, or charge nurse	The prudent nurse knows when to seek assistance.	b. Tidy the bed and unit, place call light and personal items within reach, and provide for safety by raising the siderails and lowering the bed	
• Strive for efficiency of time and effort within the framework of delivering safe care	Work organization and time efficiency are important when caring for a group of patients.	c. Place soiled linens in the correct hamper	Contaminated items must be contained or cleaned in order to prevent the spread of microorganisms
At the end of the procedure:		d. Clean reusable items and return to storage or processing area (Central Supply)	
X. Remove gloves and other protective gear and wash hands	Contaminated gloves and coverings might contaminate other objects or people.	e. Stop equipment charges	Patients should not be charged for equipment they are no longer using

IMPORTANT STEPS	KEY POINTS/RATIONALE	IMPORTANT STEPS	KEY POINTS/RATIONALE
Y. (*continued*)		**Z.** Record and report the procedure:	All procedures must be documented.
f. Remove potentially infectious trash from the room		a. Document assessment findings and details of the procedure performed, or care given, in the chart. Include any problems encountered	
g. Provide necessary teaching related to the procedure performed	Learning is reinforced when teaching is accompanied by a demonstration.		Problems must be documented.
h. Inquire if anything else is needed	Prevents having to return to the room in the immediate future.	b. Record the data concisely and accurately; be specific rather than general	Data recorded should present a "picture" of what occurred.
i. Re-wash hands before leaving the room	Hands must be re-washed after handling soiled equipment and trash.	c. Report abnormalities to the charge nurse or physician as need indicates	Abnormalities must be reported so that action, if needed, can be taken to correct the situation.

Chapter 1

Legal, Ethical and Financial Considerations in Clinical Nursing

LEARNING ACTIVITIES

I. Define and give an example of each of the following terms:

1. standard of care

2. negligence

3. malpractice

4. civil law

5. criminal law

6. invasion of privacy

7. slander

8. assault and battery

© 1994 W.B. Saunders Company. *Rambo's Nursing Skills for Clinical Practice,* fourth edition
All rights reserved.

II. Ways in which nurses can prevent client law suits against themselves or the hospital include:

*III. **Matching.** For each of the patients listed in Column 1, select the category of person from Column 2 who must sign the consent form or legally give consent for the medical treatment.*

Column 1

_____ 1. A woman, age 38, married, who is unconscious from an overdose of a tranquilizer.

_____ 2. A girl, age 17, married, with an upper respiratory infection.

_____ 3. A woman, age 22, single, mentally retarded, for breast biopsy.

_____ 4. A male, age 16, living in nearby city with friends, for abdominal pain.

_____ 5. A male, age 45, severe injuries from car accident following an evening of drinking.

_____ 6. A girl, age 14, for treatment of pregnancy.

_____ 7. A baby, 6 months old, with pneumonia.

Column 2

A. by the parent

B. by the patient for own self

C. by a guardian

D. by spouse

E. by implied consent

*IV. **Multiple Choice.** For each of the following questions, select the one best answer.*

1. Which consent form is used to show the patient has consented to have blood drawn for laboratory tests, treatments by the nurses such as dressing a wound or catheterization, and treatment by the physical or respiratory therapist?

    a. consent for surgery
    b. "informed consent"
    c. conditions of admission
    d. consent for special procedures

2. Which one of the following is NOT considered an incident and does not need to be reported on an incident or occurrence form?

    a. a fall to the floor while getting out of bed.
    b. a hole burned into the mattress from a smoldering cigarette butt.
    c. giving the patient the wrong medication.
    d. the patient's having developed a pressure area on the sacrum.

© 1994 W.B. Saunders Company. *Rambo's Nursing Skills for Clinical Practice,* fourth edition
All rights reserved.

3. What happens to the incident report after it is made out?

    a. It becomes part of the patient's chart.
    b. It is sent to Medical Records.
    c. It is sent to the Administration office.
    d. A copy is given to the patient.

V. Read the Code for Nurses and the Code of Ethics for the Licensed Practical Nurse. When you have completed your study of the two codes, fill in the following blanks:

1. a. Ethics is a code of _____ _____

    b. that represents _____conduct

    c. for a particular _____

2. A violation of ethical behavior may result in discipline by_____ or loss of_____ .

VI. Try out your new concepts of ethics by reading the following hypothetical situations and filling in the blanks or circling the appropriate italicized word or words.

Situation A

    Mr. Brown in Room 201 is in critical condition and, although you have not cared for him, you have heard one of the other nurses mention that the doctor feels the patient will not live much longer. A relative of the client asks you in the corridor if Mr. Brown has improved. Your answer might be, "You probably need to speak to the doctor about that."

1. Ethically, who is being considered here?

    a. _____

    b. _____

    c. _____

2. In any situation in which the answer is not clear to you, it is appropriate to refer the question to your _____.

3. In doing the above, you recognize your:

    a. legal limitations
    b. ethical limitations
    c. both legal and ethical limitations

Situation B

    A young girl has been brought by ambulance to the Emergency Room. You are the admitting nurse there and note that she has swallowed an overdose of sedatives and is now having her stomach emptied of its contents. Since this was an attempted suicide, the police reporters were in the hallway. When you go to lunch, your friends from other units want to know why the ambulance had its siren sounding, how old the girl is, and why she was brought in. You were the person who recorded the emergency room notes into her chart and so you have some information.

4. When asked if the girl took an overdose, you might answer:

    a. Yes, but she's O.K.
    b. She must have had a desire to die.
    c. This information is confidential.

5. In this situation, to discuss the client not only violates her right to privacy, but could result in a: _____ and possibly _____ employment.

© 1994 W.B. Saunders Company. *Rambo's Nursing Skills for Clinical Practice,* fourth edition
All rights reserved.

Situation C

Carol Brown, an LPN on your unit, has always been conscientious and reliable in her work habits. She is scheduled to work on the weekend and receives an invitation from an old friend to spend the weekend at Yosemite National Park. Carol has never been to Yosemite and does not often have such opportunities. She ponders long and hard before arriving at a decision.

6. Persons she should consider in making her decision include:

   a. _____

   b. _____

   c. _____

   d. _____

Situation D

Mr. Grimm, in the Suite at the end of the hall, always orders his meals from the hospital's special gourmet menu. At noon on Sunday he didn't touch any of the food, although the meal was excellent. The chef salad and strawberry pie were tempting to you. You pick up his tray from his room.

7. Thinking that it is a shame to waste such food, you:

   a. give it to the housekeeping staff.
   b. send it back to the kitchen.
   c. offer it to the entire unit staff.
   d. eat it yourself.

Situation E

A unit secretary is very tense about her new job on the cardiac telemetry unit. Her doctor has prescribed a mild tranquilizer for her. She knows that when clients go home, the medications are often left behind and returned to the pharmacy. She asks the nurses if they could give her the tranquilizers that are left upon a patient's discharge, saving her the expense of having the prescription filled.

8. This is a distinct breach of _____ on her part.

9. If the nurses grant her request, they are prescribing or dispensing medicine without a license and this is a _____ offense.

Situation F

You have been Mrs. Johann's nurse for her entire stay in the hospital. She has come to rely on you and, when she is ready to go home, wants to give you a sum of money in appreciation for the "lovely things you have done for her."

10. In this situation you should:

   a. explain to her that the service is part of her care.
   b. accept the money because, although you receive a salary from the hospital, clients should pay for the service you render them individually.
   c. accept the gift of money and tell nobody so that no one else will feel hurt that she selected only you.
   d. suggest she give the money to the health aide who needs it more than you do.

11. Mrs. Johann insists that you take the money or you will hurt her feelings. Therefore you:

   a. tell her of some specific need the hospital has to which she could make a contribution.
   b. suggest a fund in her name with suitable recognition.
   c. accept the gift so that there are no hurt feelings in the situation.
   d. tell her to give it to the health aide since she needs the money more than you do.

12. The functions and boundaries of nursing practice are legally defined in:

   a. the Code for Nurses
   b. the hospital Procedure Manual
   c. the Standards of Nursing Care
   d. the state Nursing Practice Act

13. The purpose of the Standards of Nursing Practice is to

   _____

   _____

   and to _____

14. One method of determining whether standards of nursing care are being met in a hospital is the performance of a _____ .

15. As long as a nurse follows her agency's Policy and Procedure Manual, she will be giving an accepted _____ .

16. The Medicare reimbursement system is based on DRGs which means that the fees for services are paid by _____ based on the client's diagnosis.

VII. Take the post-test included at the end of the chapter in the text.

© 1994 W.B. Saunders Company. *Rambo's Nursing Skills for Clinical Practice,* fourth edition
All rights reserved.

PERFORMANCE CHECKLIST

Skill 1-1   Procedure for obtaining a signature

Student: _____

Date: _____

	Satisfactory	**Unsatisfactory**
1. Carries out Standard Steps A, B, C, D, and E as need indicates.	❏	❏
2. Obtains correct form and fills in patient name, age, sex, room, physician, procedure, and date.	❏	❏
3. Has patient read over the form allowing time for questions.	❏	❏
4. Determines whether patient is "informed" (understands the procedure, potential complications, ramifications and risks).	❏	❏
5. Witnesses patient signing the form.	❏	❏
6. In the event the person refuses to sign the form, reports to the charge nurse and notifies the physician.	❏	❏
7. Signs the form on the witness line with full name and title.	❏	❏
8. Places the completed form in the patient's chart.	❏	❏

Pass _____

Fail _____

Comments: _____

_____

Instructor: _____

© 1994 W.B. Saunders Company. *Rambo's Nursing Skills for Clinical Practice,* fourth edition
All rights reserved.

PERFORMANCE CHECKLIST

Skill 1-2 Incident report

Student: _____

Date: _____

	Satisfactory	Unsatisfactory
1. Provides for the person's safety and comfort.	❑	❑
2. Notifies the physician of the occurrence if a patient is involved.	❑	❑
3. Carries out the physician's orders.	❑	❑
4. Obtains factual account of the occurrence.	❑	❑
5. Fills out incident report form.	❑	❑
6. Distributes the form according to agency protocol.	❑	❑
7. Monitors person's status as need requires.	❑	❑

Pass _____

Fail _____

Comments: _____

_____

Instructor: _____

© 1994 W.B. Saunders Company. *Rambo's Nursing Skills for Clinical Practice*, fourth edition
All rights reserved.

SUGGESTED CLINICAL ACTIVITIES

The following activities may enhance your learning and retention of the material in chapter one.

1. Review the documentation in the nurse's notes for one of your assigned patients from the previous 24 hours. Determine if you feel that it meets the guidelines for legally sound charting. Look at legibility, judgmental statements, objectivity, thoroughness, correction of any errors. Are there any problems noted for which interventions do not seem to have been done? Think about how you might have charted differently.

2. During a clinical day, observe for ways in which patient's rights are being observed. Were there any instances of when patient's rights were violated? Discuss these in your clinical group.

© 1994 W.B. Saunders Company. *Rambo's Nursing Skills for Clinical Practice,* fourth edition
All rights reserved.

Chapter 2

Basic Medical Terminology

LEARNING ACTIVITIES

EXERCISE 1

DIRECTIONS: Divide each of the following medical terms into its basic elements and translate the term. Use a nursing or medical dictionary for any unfamiliar terms.

1. Hysterosalpingectomy *Hystero/salping/ectomy* removal of the uterus.

2. Gastroenteritis _____

3. Intravenous _____

4. Appendicitis _____

5. Angiocardiopathy _____

EXERCISE 2

DIRECTIONS: Find the root of the following words and give the meaning of the terms.

1. Adenoma   *aden*   tumor of a gland

2. Dyspepsia _____

3. Pathogenic _____

4. Antidote _____

5. Toxic _____

EXERCISE 3

DIRECTIONS: Give the correct meaning for each of the following abbreviations.

1. qd _____

2. c _____

3. PRN _____

4. ad lib _____

5. BP _____

6. STAT _____

7. OS _____

8. I & O _____

9. BRP _____

10. RUQ _____

EXERCISE 4

DIRECTIONS: Match the abbreviations, acronyms, and symbols in Column 1 with the correct label from Column 2.

	Term		Label
1. ___	ANA	a.	Abbreviation
2. ___	>	b.	Acronym
3. ___	ml	c.	Symbol
4. ___	H		
5. ___	CDC		
6. ___	o		
7. ___	℥		
8. ___	CAP		
9. ___	L		
10. ___	"		

EXERCISE 5

Multiple Choice: Choose the best answer for the following questions:

1. 2 tabs q.o.d. p.o. tells the nurse to give the patient:

   a. 2 tablets every day after dinner.
   b. 2 tablets four times a day by mouth.
   c. 2 tablets every other day before meals.
   d. 2 tablets every other day by mouth.

2. If an order for drop-type medications states 1 drop "O.S." every 8 hours, it means:

   a. place 1 drop in the right eye every 8 hours.
   b. place a drop in the left eye every 8 hours.
   c. place one drop in each eye every 8 hours.
   d. place one drop in the left ear every 8 hours.

3. An order reading "BRP" means:

   a. bathroom privileges.
   b. bed rest preferred.
   c. by peripheral route.
   d. bottom rail permitted down.

4. "PRN" attached to an order means that the order may be done:

   a. by an RN only.
   b. preferably right now.
   c. as needed.
   d. permitted rest needed.

EXERCISE 6

Take the post-test included at the end of the chapter in the text.

SUGGESTED CLINICAL ACTIVITIES

1. Scan through the history and physical of an assigned patient and jot down terms that are unfamiliar. Look up the terms in a medical dictionary. Share your new knowledge with a classmate.

2. Read an article in a current nursing journal; note any unfamiliar terms and look them up in a medical dictionary.

3. Bring one new term per clinical day back to conference and share the term and its meaning with your classmates.

© 1994 W.B. Saunders Company. *Rambo's Nursing Skills for Clinical Practice,* fourth edition
All rights reserved.

Chapter 3

Communication and the Nurse-Patient Relationship

LEARNING ACTIVITIES

I. Fill in the blanks.

1. Communication consists of both _____ and _____ behaviors.

2. The expression of thoughts or emotions by means of posture of gestures is called _____.

3. Information that a patient reveals to a nurse must be kept _____.

4. For a communication to be complete, the speaker must receive _____.

5. Five factors that affect the way a person communicates are: _____, _____, _____, _____ and _____.

II. For the following communication techniques, indicate with a checkmark which ones are considered non-therapeutic (blocks to communication).

1. Silence _____

2. Reflection _____

3. Interrupting _____

4. Agreeing _____

5. Clarifying _____

6. Changing the subject _____

7. Offering self _____

8. Offering false reassurance _____

9. Questioning _____

10. Giving advice _____

11. General leads _____

12. Restatement _____

13. Judgmental responses _____

14. Probing questions _____

15. Open-ended questions _____

16. Giving information _____

17. Looking at alternatives _____

18. Encouraging elaboration _____

19. Using cliches _____

20. Defensive comments _____

21. Summarizing _____

22. Inattentive listening _____

© 1994 W.B. Saunders Company. *Rambo's Nursing Skills for Clinical Practice,* fourth edition   13
All rights reserved.

III. From the following scenario, underline the information that should be included in the end-of-shift report.

Mr. Flicker, room 328, states he is in pain and wants his medication. At 8:30 a.m. he is given a Vicodan. The pain was relieved by 9:15. He was interrupted by three phone calls during his assisted bath. His IV site is clean and dry; the doctor discontinued the IV when he made afternoon rounds. The dressing over the abdominal incision is clean and dry. His wife came to visit at noon. He is cooperative with his coughing and deep breathing exercises. He walked in the hall three times. He has been taking fluids and a clear liquid diet without signs of nausea. IV. Match the communication technique in column two with the type of communication listed in column one.

IV. Matching

Column 1	**Column 2**
_____ 1. "... won't do it?"	a. Offering self
_____ 2. "...go on .."	b. clarifying
_____ 3. "He said you couldn't go home until Saturday."	c. restatement
_____ 4. "I'll come quickly if you call."	d. summarizing
_____ 5. "So, you have pain when you move, but it isn't very bad."	e. using silence
_____ 6. Leaning forward, nodding head...	f. giving information
_____ 7. "How do you feel about that?"	g. open ended question
_____ 8. "Tell me what the doctor said."	h. general lead
_____ 9. "You think it was the coffee that kept you awake?"	i. reflection
_____ 10. "Your surgery is scheduled for 10:00 a.m."	

V. Take the post-test included at the end of the chapter in the text.

© 1994 W.B. Saunders Company. *Rambo's Nursing Skills for Clinical Practice,* fourth edition
All rights reserved.

PERFORMANCE CHECKLIST

Skill 3-1   Giving end-of-shift report

Student: _____

Date: _____

	Satisfactory	Unsatisfactory
1. Efficiently organizes information for report.	❏	❏
2. Speaks clearly, enunciates, and with voice volume loud enough to be heard by all at report.	❏	❏
3. Focuses on essential information.	❏	❏
4. Identifies treatments and procedures that need to be done within next two hours.	❏	❏
5. Allows time for questions at the end of report.	❏	❏

Pass _____

Fail _____

Comments: _____

_____

Instructor: _____

© 1994 W.B. Saunders Company. *Rambo's Nursing Skills for Clinical Practice,* fourth edition
All rights reserved.

PERFORMANCE CHECKLIST

Skill 3-2 Performing a process recording

Student: _____

Date: _____

	Satisfactory	Unsatisfactory
1. Establishes rapport with patient and plans time for interaction.	❑	❑
2. Sets scene and identifies focus of recording.	❑	❑
3. Identifies patient non-verbal behaviors.	❑	❑
4. Relates patient's verbal statements in sequence.	❑	❑
5. Identifies own non-verbal behaviors.	❑	❑
6. Relates own verbal statements in sequence.	❑	❑
7. Labels own statements as to whether it was therapeutic or non-therapeutic.	❑	❑
8. When a non-therapeutic comment is identified, notes statement that would have been more therapeutic under the circumstances.	❑	❑

Pass _____

Fail _____

Comments: _____

_____

Instructor: _____

© 1994 W.B. Saunders Company. *Rambo's Nursing Skills for Clinical Practice,* fourth edition
All rights reserved.

Suggested Clinical Activities

1. Listen carefully to various nurses give report. Determine which one gives the best report and try and figure out why you feel this report is the best.

2. When you come home from your clinical experience, take the information you have on your work sheet for the patients you cared for and using a tape recorder, practice giving report.

3. Plan a specific interaction with a family member and practice using therapeutic communication techniques.

4. During lunch, practice "attentive" listening with a classmate.

5. Review your interactions with patients on the way home at the end of the clinical day. Pick out any instances where you felt your communication was ineffective and by using therapeutic techniques, see what you could have said that might have made the outcome of the interaction better.

© 1994 W.B. Saunders Company. *Rambo's Nursing Skills for Clinical Practice,* fourth edition
All rights reserved.

Chapter 4

Application of the Nursing Process

LEARNING ACTIVITIES

I. Fill in the blanks.

1. In order to perform even the simplest nursing skill you need to _____ how to do it.

2. Whenever nursing care is performed, it is essential to consider the _____ needs of the patient.

3. A nursing data base is compiled by using the _____ process.

4. What nursing problems are present for a patient is determined by _____ the assessment data.

5. In most agencies, nursing problems of the patient are stated as nursing _____.

6. Nursing care is delivered by considering the order of _____ of the patient's needs or problems.

7. Outcome statements should be written so that it is easy to _____ whether they have been met or not.

8. When formulating a nursing care plan, the nurse chooses interventions that are most likely to meet the _____.

9. In order to function effectively, the nurse must use a method of _____.

10. To determine whether the nursing care plan is effective, the nurse _____ the effect of the interventions.

© 1994 W.B. Saunders Company. *Rambo's Nursing Skills for Clinical Practice,* fourth edition   21
All rights reserved.

II. Determine which outcome/goal statements are long-term and which are short-term; label each one accordingly.

1. Patient will walk to the end of the hall three times a day.

2. Patient will establish a 30 minute, 3 times a week exercise program.

3. Patient will regain use of right hand as evidenced by ability to tie shoes.

4. Patient will participate in physical therapy twice a day this week.

5. Patient will adhere to fluid restrictions as evidenced by intake record.

6. Patient will maintain a weight loss of two pounds a month over the next 12 months.

III. Determine which data is subjective and which is objective. Write an "S" or an "O" beside each one to indicate your choice.

____ 1. Blood pressure 128/78

____ 2. States feels tired.

____ 3. Rash on right forearm.

____ 4. Sleeping at intervals.

____ 5. Has headache.

____ 6. Lungs clear to auscultation.

____ 7. "I think I have fever".

____ 8. Skin hot to touch.

____ 9. Winces when abdomen is palpated.

____ 10. Complains of itching.

IV. List four different methods you can use in assessing the patient.

_____

_____

_____

_____

V. Place the numbers 1 through 6 in the blanks in the usual order of the steps for performing a nursing task.

_____ Clean and dispose of used supplies.

_____ Document.

_____ Prepare the patient.

_____ Explain the procedure.

_____ Restore the unit and make the patient comfortable.

_____ Perform the procedure.

© 1994 W.B. Saunders Company. *Rambo's Nursing Skills for Clinical Practice,* fourth edition
All rights reserved.

VI. Identify nursing diagnoses that seem likely to be correct for the following patients:

1. Mrs. Anderson is admitted with severe abdominal pain.

    _____

2. Mr. Harper has fallen and fractured his hip.

    _____

3. Johnny is admitted with burns on his chest.

    _____

4. Although recovering, Mr. Hutton suffered a stroke that has paralyzed his right extremities.

    _____

5. Mrs. Alton has emphysema and becomes very short of breath whenever she tries to perform a task.

    _____

VII. Take the post-test included at the end of the chapter in the text.

© 1994 W.B. Saunders Company. *Rambo's Nursing Skills for Clinical Practice,* fourth edition
All rights reserved.

PERFORMANCE CHECKLIST

Skill 4-1   Constructing a nursing care plan

Student: _____

Date: _____

	Satisfactory	Unsatisfactory
1. Carries out Standard Steps A, B, and C.	❏	❏
2. Adequately assesses the patient.	❏	❏
3. Carries out Standard Steps X, Y, and Z.	❏	❏
4. Recognizes or writes appropriate nursing diagnoses.**	❏	❏
5. Each nursing diagnosis is supported by appropriate data.	❏	❏
6. Lists nursing diagnoses in correct order of priority. Collaborates with patient concerning priorities.	❏	❏
7. Writes short and long-term goals/expected outcomes that are easily measured.	❏	❏
8. Plans appropriate nursing interventions for each nursing diagnosis; includes independent and dependent actions.	❏	❏
9. Implements the plan of care; documents appropriately.	❏	❏
10. Evaluates the outcome of each nursing intervention; determines if progress toward goals/expected outcomes is occurring.	❏	❏
11. Revises nursing care plan as data indicates need.	❏	❏

** LPN/LVN students recognize appropriate nursing diagnoses for the
patient. RN students write nursing diagnoses.

Pass _____

Fail _____

Comments: _____

Instructor _____

© 1994 W.B. Saunders Company. *Rambo's Nursing Skills for Clinical Practice,* fourth edition
All rights reserved.

Suggested Clinical Activities

1. Before your first clinical patient assignment, perform an assessment on a classmate, friend, or family member.

2. Review the nursing assessment and history form on your assigned patient's chart. Note the types of information and the nursing comments it contains.

3. Find the physician's history and physical on your assigned patient's chart. Read it. Look up any unfamiliar terms.

4. Perform an assessment on your assigned patient. Now find the nursing care plan in the patient's chart. Determine if the nursing diagnoses that were designated for this patient are appropriate by determining if the data you collected supports these nursing diagnoses. Are there other nursing diagnoses that would be appropriate that seem to be missing?

© 1994 W.B. Saunders Company. *Rambo's Nursing Skills for Clinical Practice,* fourth edition
All rights reserved.

Chapter 5

Handwashing, Medical Asepsis, and Universal Precautions

LEARNING ACTIVITIES

I. Fill in the blanks with the correct words.

1. The single most important aspect of using medical asepsis is *handwashing*.

2. Medical asepsis is very important in the prevention of the spread of *microorganisms*

3. Pathogens are microorganisms capable of spreading *infection*.

4. Microorganisms are spread by the following four routes:

    a. *Direct + Indirect*

    b. *Vehicle*

    c. *Air*

    d. *Vector (tick)*

5. The most common method of transmitting microorganisms within the health care setting is by *direct contact w/ an infected person*.

6. Nonpathogenic microorganisms can become pathogenic by *mutation*.

7. Microorganisms can be killed by the process of *sterilization*.

8. The severity of infection caused by microorganisms depends on

    a. _____

    b. _____

    c. _____

9. Three natural defenses of the body against infection are:

    a. _____

    b. _____

    c. _____

10. Immunity to disease can be either *natural* or *acquired* .

11. Four ways to kill or control microorganisms are:

    a. *disinfection*

    b. *Steam under pressure*

    c. *Isolation*

    d. *Handwashing w/ Soap & Water*

12. The two viruses that brought about the formulation of the universal precaution guidelines are:

    a. _____

    b. _____

13. Universal precautions involve using safe practices for protection from exposure to

    _____ .

14. Universal precautions require that all patients by treated as if _____ .

15. Barriers, called _____ are used by health care workers to protect themselves and other patients from the transmission of blood borne organisms.

16. Hands should be washed for _____ seconds between patients.

17. The only jewelry that should be worn when working with patients is

    _____ .

© 1994 W.B. Saunders Company. *Rambo's Nursing Skills for Clinical Practice,* fourth edition
All rights reserved.

18. After performing a handwash the faucets should be turned off by using a _____ unless there is an elbow or knee control.

19. When there is a possibility of splashing of body fluids, the nurse must don

_____ .

20. Gloves are to be used anytime there is a possibility that the nurse's hands may come in contact with

_____ .

II. Match the term in Column II with the definition in Column I.

____ 1. anaerobic
____ 2. antiseptic
____ 3. asepsis
____ 4. debris
____ 5. pathogenic
____ 6. sterile
____ 7. unsterile
____ 8. contaminate

a. contaminated with living microorganisms.
b. causing infection.
c. free from living microorganisms.
d. to render unclean or unsterile
e. anything which lives or grows in the absence of oxygen.
f. preventing or arresting the growth or action of microorganisms.
g. dead tissue or foreign matter.
h. anything that requires oxygen to live and grow.
i. freedom from infection or infectious material.
j. infections acquired during hospitalization.

III. Take the post-test included at the end of the chapter in the text.

© 1994 W.B. Saunders Company. *Rambo's Nursing Skills for Clinical Practice,* fourth edition
All rights reserved.

PERFORMANCE CHECKLIST

Skill 5-1   Handwashing

Student: _____

Date: _____

	Satisfactory	Unsatisfactory
1. Stands away from sink to prevent contaminating uniform.	❑	❑
2. Uses constantly running water.	❑	❑
3. Wets hands.	❑	❑
4. Soaps hands sufficiently to provide lather.	❑	❑
5. Washes entire surfaces of hands and wrists using friction.	❑	❑
6. Interlaces fingers to wash spaces between them; rubs back and forth.	❑	❑
7. Washes for at least 30 seconds.	❑	❑
8. Rinses hands well with fingers pointing down.	❑	❑
9. Dries hands thoroughly.	❑	❑
10. Turns off water without contaminating hands.	❑	❑

Pass _____

Fail _____

Comments: _____

_____

Instructor: _____

© 1994 W.B. Saunders Company. *Rambo's Nursing Skills for Clinical Practice,* fourth edition
All rights reserved.

Suggested Clinical Activities

1. Locate areas where clean disposable gloves are kept so that you can replenish the container in a patient's room as needed.

2. Locate other items of personal protective equipment including masks, impermeable gowns, and eye wear, on your assigned unit.

3. Practice the handwash procedure several times at home; try to always wash your hands in this manner so that it will become an automatic procedure.

4. For one hour on your assigned nursing unit, observe for breaks in the use of medical asepsis and universal precautions. Discuss what you observed in clinical conference with your peers.

© 1994 W.B. Saunders Company. *Rambo's Nursing Skills for Clinical Practice,* fourth edition
All rights reserved.

Chapter 6

Body Alignment and Maintenance of Musculoskeletal Function

LEARNING ACTIVITIES

I. Fill in the blanks with the most appropriate answer.

1. List five movements that you might perform in your daily hospital work.

   a. _____

   b. _____

   c. _____

   d. _____

   e. _____

2. Give three reasons for using good body alignment, balance, and movement.

   a. _____

   b. _____

   c. _____

3. A very common injury among hospital workers is _____.

4. A force that pulls any object toward the ground is called _____.

5. Pick up your heaviest book or a similar object and hold it out at arm's length for at least 30 seconds. Now bring it close to your body for the same length of time.

   a. What difference did you notice in its apparent weight? _____

   _____

   b. Explain why this is so. _____

6. List three methods you might use in order to work at a comfortable height.

   a. _____

   b. _____

   c. _____

7. How might you avoid hyperextending your back if you were asked to support a patient's leg in a cast while the doctor

   worked on the cast? _____

8. Why is it best to "set" or prepare the muscles before performing a strenuous activity? _____

   _____

9. Why is leverage important? _____

   _____

10. What causes resistance to movement? _____

11. How do you provide lateral stability when reaching? _____

12. Why would you shift your weight to the ball of each foot before making the pivoting turn? _____

    _____

13. List two nursing activities in which a pivoting turn could be used to prevent twisting the trunk of the body.

    a. _____

    b. _____

14. When carrying an object, why is it best to hold it close to your body? _____

15. List three ways to reduce strain if you must lift and carry heavy objects.

    a. _____

    b. _____

    c. _____

© 1994 W.B. Saunders Company. *Rambo's Nursing Skills for Clinical Practice*, fourth edition
All rights reserved.

16. List two safety precautions to observe if you are pushing or pulling a stretcher with a patient on it in the hospital corridor.

   a. _____

   b. _____

17. What do you do in pushing an object that utilizes your body weight as an additional force? _____

   _____

18. Four reasons for changing the position of the patient are:

   a. _____

   b. _____

   c. _____

   d. _____

19. When the bed patient is positioned by the nurse, it is necessary to maintain _____

   _____.

20. The discomfort felt by the patient when lying in one position for a long period of time is the result of _____

   _____ .

21. Name four of the areas where discomfort may be felt when a person is lying in the supine position.

   a. _____

   b. _____

   c. _____

   d. _____

22. Two reasons for using aids in positioning the patient are:

   a. _____

   b. _____

23. The effects of pressure on the lungs lead to the complication of _____.

24. Pressure areas on the skin most often develop over _____ of bones.

© 1994 W.B. Saunders Company. *Rambo's Nursing Skills for Clinical Practice,* fourth edition
All rights reserved.

25. The first sign of pressure usually noticed by the nurse is _____ of the skin.

26. The primary method used by hospital workers to prevent the formation of pressure areas in the bed patient is

    _____.

27. In addition to the primary method, wheat other two methods might you use for the patient who shows signs of pressure on the skin over his sacrum?

    a. _____

    b. _____

28. The four principles used in positioning the helpless bed patient are:

    a. _____

    b. _____

    c. _____

    d. _____

II. Take the post-test included at the end of the chapter in the text.

© 1994 W.B. Saunders Company. *Rambo's Nursing Skills for Clinical Practice,* fourth edition
All rights reserved.

PERFORMANCE CHECKLIST

Skill 6-1   Moving a patient up in bed

Student: _____

Date: _____

		Satisfactory	**Unsatisfactory**
1.	Carries out Standard Steps A, B, C, D, and E as indicated.	❏	❏
2.	Positions bed: locks wheels, raises bed to correct working height in flat position, lowers near side-rail, removes pillows.	❏	❏
3.	Instructs patient if patient can assist.	❏	❏
4.	Positions patient with knees flexed and arms across chest if patient is unable to help.	❏	❏
5.	Shifts patient up in bed using proper body mechanics.	❏	❏

FOR LIFT (DRAW) SHEET:

6.	Obtains assistant to help.	❏	❏
7.	Places lift (draw) sheet under patient, fan-folded close to patient.	❏	❏
8.	On count of three both nurses slide lift sheet and patient toward head of bed using correct body mechanics.	❏	❏
9.	Carries out Standard Steps X, Y, and Z.	❏	❏

Pass _____

Fail _____

Comments: _____

_____

Instructor: _____

© 1994 W.B. Saunders Company. *Rambo's Nursing Skills for Clinical Practice,* fourth edition
All rights reserved.

PERFORMANCE CHECKLIST

Skill 6-2   Placing the patient in the supine position

Student: _____

Date: _____

	Satisfactory	**Unsatisfactory**
1. Carries out Standard Steps A, B, C, D, and E as indicated.	❏	❏
2. Prepares bed: proper working height, bed flat, near side-rail down, wheels locked.	❏	❏
3. Places patient's body in good alignment.	❏	❏
4. Positions pillows under head and shoulders and a small pillow or roll under the knees.	❏	❏
5. Uses footboard and trochanter rolls as need indicates.	❏	❏
6. Places pillow or padding between the knees and positions arms and supports with pillows.	❏	❏
7. Positions hands in proper alignment using supports or splints as need indicates.	❏	❏
8. Carries out Standard Steps X, Y, and Z.	❏	❏

Pass _____

Fail _____

Comments: _____

_____

Instructor: _____

© 1994 W.B. Saunders Company. *Rambo's Nursing Skills for Clinical Practice,* fourth edition
All rights reserved.

PERFORMANCE CHECKLIST

Skill 6-3 Placing the patient in a Fowler's or Semi-Fowler's Position

Student: _____

Date: _____

	Satisfactory	**Unsatisfactory**
1. Carries out Standard Steps A, B, C, D, and E as indicated.	❑	❑

FOWLER'S POSITION

	Satisfactory	**Unsatisfactory**
2. Elevates the head of the bed to an angle of 60–90 degrees for a high-Fowler's position or 30 - 60 degrees for a Fowler's position.	❑	❑

SEMI-FOWLER'S POSITION

	Satisfactory	**Unsatisfactory**
3. Elevates the head of the bed to an angle of 15–30 degrees for a low-Fowler's position.	❑	❑
4. Places the body in proper alignment, using pillows and supportive devices as need indicates.	❑	❑
5. Carries out Standard Steps X, Y, and Z.	❑	❑

Pass _____

Fail _____

Comments: _____

_____

Instructor: _____

© 1994 W.B. Saunders Company. *Rambo's Nursing Skills for Clinical Practice,* fourth edition
All rights reserved.

PERFORMANCE CHECKLIST

Skill 6-4 Moving the patient to the side of the bed and logrolling

Student: _____

Date: _____

	Satisfactory	Unsatisfactory
1. Carries out Standard Steps A, B, C, D, and E as indicated.	❏	❏
2. Prepares the bed: locks wheels, raises bed to proper working height, removes pillows, lowers near side-rail.	❏	❏
3. Places patient's arms across the chest.	❏	❏
4. Uses proper body mechanics, with arms as levers, and a rocking motion, to pull patient to side of the bed, starting at shoulders, then waist, then legs.	❏	❏

LOGROLLING:

	Satisfactory	Unsatisfactory
5. Obtains assistance of two more nurses or assistants.	❏	❏
6. Three nurses/assistants on the count of three, move the patient to the side of the bed as one unit, keeping the patient's spine in correct alignment.	❏	❏
7. All three nurses move to the other side of the bed after raising the side-rail.	❏	❏
8. With near side-rail lowered and pillow placed between the patient's legs and a pillow under the patient's head, three nurses position their hands and arms correctly and on the count of three, roll the patient in a smooth, even motion, keeping the patient's body in straight alignment, onto the side.	❏	❏
7. Places in desired position, checking body alignment when finished.	❏	❏
8. Carries out Standard Steps X, Y, and Z.	❏	❏

Pass _____

Fail _____

Comments: _____

_____

Instructor: _____

© 1994 W.B. Saunders Company. *Rambo's Nursing Skills for Clinical Practice,* fourth edition
All rights reserved.

PERFORMANCE CHECKLIST

Skill 6-5   Turning the patient to a lateral, prone, and supine position

Student: _____

Date: _____

	Satisfactory	Unsatisfactory
1. Carries out Standard Steps A, B, C, D, and E as indicated.	❏	❏
2. Positions the bed correctly: locks wheels, places bed flat raises bed to proper working height, removes pillows; lowers near side rail.	❏	❏

LATERAL OR MODIFIED LATERAL POSITION

	Satisfactory	Unsatisfactory
3. Moves patient to the side of the bed and raises near side-rail.	❏	❏
4. Moves to opposite side of the bed, lowers side-rail, places patient's arms across the chest.	❏	❏
5. Flexes the patient's distal knee across proximal thigh.	❏	❏
6. Using proper body mechanics and placement of hands and arms, rolls the patient onto side toward self with a smooth motion.	❏	❏
7. Positions patient in proper body alignment, using pillows and supportive devices as needed.	❏	❏
8. Supports extremities and joints when lifting them for positioning.	❏	❏

SIMS' POSITION (LEFT SEMI-PRONE)

	Satisfactory	Unsatisfactory
9. Flexes patient's upper thigh and knee toward the chest, and flexes other leg slightly; positions legs so they are not touching.	❏	❏
10. Places lower arm to the back of the patient with elbow slightly flexed.	❏	❏
11. Flexes upper arm away from the body and supports it with a pillow.	❏	❏
12. Places a small pillow under the head.	❏	❏

PRONE POSITION

	Satisfactory	Unsatisfactory
13. With patient supine, places both arms at the sides and distal ankle over proximal ankle.	❏	❏
14. Moves patient to the side of the bed.	❏	❏
15. Raises side-rail and moves to opposite side of bed; lowers near side-rail.	❏	❏
16. Rolls patient onto side, then onto abdomen, toward self.	❏	❏
17. Positions patient's head to one side with body in proper alignment.	❏	❏
18. Positions arms and legs in proper alignment.	❏	❏

© 1994 W.B. Saunders Company. *Rambo's Nursing Skills for Clinical Practice,* fourth edition
All rights reserved.

19. Places small pillow or folded towel under the head and under the chest and abdomen between the breasts for the female, and under the lower abdomen for the male.   ❏   ❏

SUPINE POSITION

20. From the prone position, places patient's head in direction opposite to which turn is to be made.   ❏   ❏

21. Places distal ankle over the other ankle.   ❏   ❏

22. Moves patient to the side of the bed opposite to the direction in which the turn will be made.   ❏   ❏

23. Raises side-rail and moves to opposite side of the bed; lowers near side-rail.   ❏   ❏

24. With proper hand and arm position, and using proper body mechanics, rolls the patient to a lateral and then supine position.   ❏   ❏

25. Places the patient's body in proper alignment, using supportive devices and pillows as need indicates.   ❏   ❏

26. Carries out Standard Steps X, Y, and Z.   ❏   ❏

Pass _____

Fail _____

Comments: _____

_____

Instructor: _____

© 1994 W.B. Saunders Company. *Rambo's Nursing Skills for Clinical Practice,* fourth edition
All rights reserved.

PERFORMANCE CHECKLIST

Skill 6-6   Range of motion exercises

Student: _____

Date: _____

	Satisfactory	Unsatisfactory
1. Carries out Standard Steps A, B, C, D, and E as indicated.	☐	☐
2. Prepares the bed: wheels locked, bed at proper working height.	☐	☐
3. Positions patient in supine position and drapes.	☐	☐
4. Performs passive range of motion exercises for the head and neck.	☐	☐
5. Performs passive range of motion on the near upper extremity, using correct movements and appropriate number of repetitions:		
A. Neck	☐	☐
B. Arm flexion, extension	☐	☐
C. Shoulder abduction, adduction, internal rotation, external rotation.	☐	☐
D. Elevation and depression of shoulders.	☐	☐
E. Wrist	☐	☐
F. Fingers	☐	☐
6. Performs passive range of motion on the near lower extremity, using correct movements and appropriate number of repetitions:		
A. Leg flexion and extension.	☐	☐
B. Hip abduction and adduction.	☐	☐
C. Hip internal rotation and external rotation.	☐	☐
D. Ankle	☐	☐
E. Foot dorsiflexion and plantar flexion	☐	☐
F. Toes	☐	☐
7. Raises side rail; moves to opposite side of bed.	☐	☐
8. Lowers side rail and performs passive ROM to upper extremity.	☐	☐
9. Perform passive ROM to lower extremity.	☐	☐
10. Places patient in position of comfort.	☐	☐
11. Carries out Standard Steps X, Y, and Z.	☐	☐

Pass _____

Fail _____

Comments: _____

_____

Instructor: _____

© 1994 W.B. Saunders Company. *Rambo's Nursing Skills for Clinical Practice,* fourth edition
All rights reserved.

PERFORMANCE CHECKLIST

Skill 6-7   Assisting the patient to sit on the side of the bed

Student: _____

Date: _____

	Satisfactory	Unsatisfactory
1. Carries out Standard Steps A, B, C, D, and E as indicated.	❑	❑
2. Prepares bed: locks wheels, raises bed to correct working height, lowers near side-rail.	❑	❑
3. Moves patient to side of the bed.	❑	❑
4. Places bed in low position and elevates the head of the bed to 45 degrees or more.	❑	❑
5. Using correct hand and arm positions and proper body mechanics, shifts patient into a sitting position on the side of the bed with the feet supported.	❑	❑
6. Assists patient to put on robe and slippers; drapes as needed for warmth.	❑	❑
7. Moves patient to side of bed so that feet are firmly on the floor; allows several minutes of sitting.	❑	❑
8. Encourages foot and lower leg exercises while dangling.	❑	❑
9. Removes robe and slippers and drape.	❑	❑
10. Using correct arm and hand positions and proper body mechanics, pivots the patient's body back onto the bed.	❑	❑
11. Places in supine position and raises side-rail.	❑	❑
12. Carries out Standard Steps X, Y, and Z.	❑	❑

Pass _____

Fail _____

Comments: _____

_____

Instructor: _____

© 1994 W.B. Saunders Company. *Rambo's Nursing Skills for Clinical Practice,* fourth edition
All rights reserved.

PERFORMANCE CHECKLIST

Skill 6-8   Assisting the patient to sit in a chair

Student: _____

Date: _____

	Satisfactory	Unsatisfactory
1. Carries out Standard Steps A, B, C, D, and E as indicated.	❑	❑
2. Place a chair at the head of the bed; if using a wheelchair, places into locked position.	❑	❑
3. Sits patient on side of bed.	❑	❑
4. Standing in front of patient, and using proper arm and hand position and proper body mechanics, assists patient to standing position; blocks patients knees and or feet with own.	❑	❑
5. Allows patient to stand and stabilize if dizzy.	❑	❑
6. Pivots patient until directly in front of the chair with back of legs touching chair.	❑	❑
7. While bracing the patient's knees, lowers patient safely into the chair.	❑	❑
8. Adjusts body alignment as needed.	❑	❑
9. Covers legs with blanket if needed.	❑	❑
10. Carries out Standard Steps X, Y, and Z.	❑	❑

Pass _____

Fail _____

Comments: _____

_____

Instructor: _____

© 1994 W.B. Saunders Company. *Rambo's Nursing Skills for Clinical Practice,* fourth edition
All rights reserved.

PERFORMANCE CHECKLIST

Skill 6-9 Assisting the patient to ambulate

Student: _____

Date: _____

	Satisfactory	Unsatisfactory
1. Carries out Standard Steps A, B, C, D, and E as indicated.	❑	❑
2. Sits the patient on the side of the bed.	❑	❑
3. Places patient's feet firmly on the floor.	❑	❑
4. Safely assists patient to a standing position using proper body mechanics.	❑	❑
5. Allows patient to stabilize and gain balance.	❑	❑
6. Moves to patient's side and provides support.	❑	❑
7. Checks and corrects patient's posture.	❑	❑
8. Walks at patient's side, matching gait, while safely stabilizing patient.	❑	❑
9. After ambulating, walks patient to the side of the bed, positions patient with legs at edge of mattress and while facing patient, assists patient to safely sit on side of bed.	❑	❑
10. Assists patient to swing feet and legs into the bed.	❑	❑
11. Assists patient to position of comfort, maintaining proper body alignment.	❑	❑
12. Carries out Standard Steps X, Y, and Z.	❑	❑

Pass _____

Fail _____

Comments: _____

_____

Instructor: _____

© 1994 W.B. Saunders Company. *Rambo's Nursing Skills for Clinical Practice,* fourth edition
All rights reserved.

PERFORMANCE CHECKLIST

Skill 6-10   Breaking a patient's fall

Student: _____

Date: _____

	Satisfactory	Unsatisfactory
1. When patient begins to fall, assumes broad stance, and grasps patient's body at waist or under the axilla.	❏	❏
2. Extends near leg against the patient, bracing patient's body and slides patient down the leg to the floor while bending own knees.	❏	❏
3. Examines patient for any sign of injury sustained in the fall.	❏	❏
4. Calls for additional help to assist the patient back to bed.	❏	❏
5. Carries out Standard Steps X, Y, and Z.	❏	❏

Pass   _____

Fail   _____

Comments: _____

_____

Instructor: _____

© 1994 W.B. Saunders Company. *Rambo's Nursing Skills for Clinical Practice,* fourth edition
All rights reserved.

Suggested Clinical Activities

1. Practice principles of body alignment and movement when performing daily tasks such as carrying groceries, reaching for things on high shelves, vacuuming, picking up a child, etc.

2. With a family member or peer, practice placing the body in the various positions used for positioning the bed patient.

3. Work with another nurse on the unit to which you are assigned and learn how she utilizes pillows and other aids in positioning the patient.

© 1994 W.B. Saunders Company. *Rambo's Nursing Skills for Clinical Practice,* fourth edition
All rights reserved.

Chapter 7

Personal Hygiene and Skin Care

LEARNING ACTIVITIES

I. Matching. Choose the statement that fits the term in Column I from Column II.

Column I

_____ 1. caries
_____ 2. excoriation
_____ 3. lochia
_____ 4. sordes
_____ 5. stomatitis
_____ 6. pediculosis
_____ 7. suppuration
_____ 8. necrosis
_____ 9. gangrene
_____10. abrasion

Column II

a. collection of brown, crusty material on the mouth and teeth.
b. inflammation of the mucosa of the mouth.
c. death of tissue due to lack of circulation.
d. decay of teeth causing a defect.
e. damage to skin caused by chemicals or burns.
f. discharge from the uterus during menstruation.
g. infested with lice.
h. formation or discharge of pus.
i. death of tissue from any cause.
j. a scraping off of a layer of skin cells.
k. fungus infection of the scalp.
l. oil-secreting glands of the skin.

II. Fill in the blanks with the appropriate word(s).

1. Regular bathing of the skin prevents _____ and _____.

2. The frequency of bathing should depend on:

   a. _____

   _____

   b. _____

   _____

3. Four functions of the skin are:

   a. _____

   _____

All rights reserved.

b. _____

_____

c. _____

_____

d. _____

_____

4. The first sign of pressure on the skin is _____.

5. Compression of the skin and tissue under it decreases the supply of _____

and _____, resulting in necrosis.

6. Damage to the skin can be further aggravated by:

a. _____

b. _____

and

c. _____

7. The prevention of pressure wounds is the responsibility of _____.

8. Four ways to prevent pressure wounds are:

a. _____

b. _____

c. _____

d. _____

9. A.M. care consists of:

_____

_____

10. Oral care is especially important for the patient receiving _____ or
radiation to the head or neck.

11. Mouth care for the unconscious patient should be performed at least once every _____ hours.

© 1994 W.B. Saunders Company. *Rambo's Nursing Skills for Clinical Practice,* fourth edition
All rights reserved.

12. When cleaning dentures, the nurse must take precautions not to _____ .

13. Four reasons for giving the patient a bath are:

    a. _____

    b. _____

    c. _____

    d. _____

14. When assisting patients with the bath, the nurse should insure that the patient does not become _____

_____ .

15. Perineal care is especially important for the female patient confined to be who is _____ .

16. Brushing and combing the hair is important because _____

_____ .

17. Hair care is usually given _____ or

_____ .

18. When shaving a patient with a safety razor, small strokes are made with the razor in the direction

_____ .

19. Before trimming the toenails, the feet should be _____ _____ .

20. When not in use, a hearing aid should be _____ .

21. P. M. care consists of _____ .

22. An important factor in providing hygiene care for each patient is that it gives the nurse an opportunity

for _____ and _____ .

23. Skin assessment should be performed at least _____ and is

also done every time _____ .

© 1994 W.B. Saunders Company. *Rambo's Nursing Skills for Clinical Practice,* fourth edition
All rights reserved.

24. When the nurse is finished with hygiene care, the unit is restored to order and the bed is returned to

   _____.

25. Besides raising the appropriate side rails, another safety factor the nurse attends to after hygiene care is to place the

   _____ within reach.

III. Take the post-test included at the end of the chapter in the text.

© 1994 W.B. Saunders Company. *Rambo's Nursing Skills for Clinical Practice,* fourth edition
All rights reserved.

PERFORMANCE CHECK LIST

Skill 7-1   Mouth care for the conscious patient

Student: _____

Date: _____

	Satisfactory	Unsatisfactory
1. Washes hands.	❑	❑
2. Uses clean gloves.	❑	❑
3. Organizes equipment.	❑	❑
4. Assesses condition of mouth.	❑	❑
5. Brushes all surfaces of all teeth.	❑	❑
6. Rinses mouth well.	❑	❑
7. Assists with flossing of teeth.	❑	❑
8. Rinses mouth.	❑	❑
9. Cleans equipment and places in storage location.	❑	❑
10. Removes gloves and washes hands.	❑	❑
11. Documents procedure on flow sheet or in nurse's notes.	❑	❑

Pass _____

Fail _____

Comments: _____

_____

Instructor: _____

© 1994 W.B. Saunders Company. *Rambo's Nursing Skills for Clinical Practice,* fourth edition
All rights reserved.

PERFORMANCE CHECKLIST

Skill 7-2 Mouth care for the unconscious patient

Student: _____

Date: _____

		Satisfactory	Unsatisfactory
1.	Washes hands.	❏	❏
2.	Attaches oral suction device to tubing and turns on suction.	❏	❏
3.	Turns patient onto side.	❏	❏
4.	Inspects inside of mouth.	❏	❏
5.	Cleanses mouth and teeth thoroughly.	❏	❏
6.	Rinses mouth	❏	❏
7.	Flosses teeth.	❏	❏
8.	Rinses mouth.	❏	❏
7.	Lubricates lips.	❏	❏
8.	Cleans and stores equipment.	❏	❏
9.	Documents procedure.	❏	❏

Pass _____

Fail _____

Comments: _____

_____

Instructor: _____

© 1994 W.B. Saunders Company. *Rambo's Nursing Skills for Clinical Practice,* fourth edition
All rights reserved.

PERFORMANCE CHECKLIST

Skill 7-3 Cleaning dentures

Student: _____

Date: _____

	Satisfactory	Unsatisfactory
1. Washes hands and dons clean gloves.	❏	❏
2. Removes dentures and places in emesis basin.	❏	❏
3. Places washcloth or towels in bottom of sink.	❏	❏
4. Cleans dentures thoroughly.	❏	❏
5. Rinses dentures.	❏	❏
6. Replaces dentures in mouth or stores in denture cup with fresh water.	❏	❏
7. Removes gloves and washes hands.	❏	❏
8. Documents procedure.	❏	❏

Pass _____

Fail _____

Comments: _____

_____

Instructor: _____

© 1994 W.B. Saunders Company. *Rambo's Nursing Skills for Clinical Practice,* fourth edition
All rights reserved.

PERFORMANCE CHECKLIST

Skill 7-4 Giving a complete bed bath

Student: _____

Date: _____

	Satisfactory	Unsatisfactory
1. Washes hands, gathers equipment, identifies patient and explains procedure.	❑	❑
2. Raises bed to working height.	❑	❑
3. Drapes patient with bath blanket or top sheet.	❑	❑
4. Removes bed linen and disposes of soiled linen not to be reused correctly.	❑	❑
5. Removes gown without exposing patient.	❑	❑
6. Washes and dries the face using separate corner of mitt for each eye.	❑	❑
7. Washes and dries the arms; protects bedding.	❑	❑
8. Washes and dries the chest using circular motions. Keeps patient draped.	❑	❑
9. Washes and dries the abdomen. Keeps patient draped.	❑	❑
10. Washes and dries the legs with long firm strokes; Places towel lengthwise under the leg.	❑	❑
11. Washes and dries the feet; soaks feet in basin.	❑	❑
12. Changes water when it becomes cool or overly soapy.	❑	❑
13. Washes and dries the back.	❑	❑
14. Gives back rub.	❑	❑
15. Washes or permits the patient to wash the perineal area; uses gloves.	❑	❑
16. Assists patient into clean gown or pajamas.	❑	❑
17. Makes occupied bed.	❑	❑
18. Removes and cleans equipment and places in storage area.	❑	❑
19. Lowers bed, raises siderails, replaces call light and tidies area.	❑	❑
20. Documents procedure.	❑	❑

Pass _____

Fail _____

Comments: _____

_____

Instructor: _____

© 1994 W.B. Saunders Company. *Rambo's Nursing Skills for Clinical Practice,* fourth edition
All rights reserved.

PERFORMANCE CHECKLIST

Skill 7-5 Partial bath

Student: _____

Date: _____

	Satisfactory	Unsatisfactory
1. Check the order, identify the patient, gather the equipment, raise the bed, and provide privacy.	❑	❑
2. Position the patient at side of bed.	❑	❑
3. Drape with bath blanket.	❑	❑
4. Remove gown.	❑	❑
5. Wash and dry the face, hands, and underarm area.	❑	❑
6. Wash and dry the genital and perianal area.	❑	❑
7. Assist patient into clean gown or pajamas.	❑	❑
8. Complete oral care, hair care and shave the male patient as needed.	❑	❑
9. Lower the bed, make patient comfortable and tidy area.	❑	❑
10. Clean and replace equipment.	❑	❑
11. Document the procedure.	❑	❑

Pass _____

Fail _____

Comments: _____

_____

Instructor: _____

© 1994 W.B. Saunders Company. *Rambo's Nursing Skills for Clinical Practice,* fourth edition
All rights reserved.

PERFORMANCE CHECKLIST

Skill 7-6   Nail care

Student: _____

Date: _____

	Satisfactory	Unsatisfactory
1. Wash hands, check orders, identify the patient, explain the procedure.	❑	❑
2. Soak the nails to soften them.	❑	❑
3. Clean under each nail; wipe nail stick on towel before cleaning next nail.	❑	❑
4. Push back cuticle on each nail.	❑	❑
5. Cut each nail straight across, even with end of finger or toe.	❑	❑
6. Dry hands and feet thoroughly.	❑	❑
7. Smooth and shape nails to contour of finger or toe.	❑	❑
8. Apply lotion to hands and feet.	❑	❑
9. Clean equipment and place in storage area.	❑	❑
10. Document procedure.	❑	❑

Pass _____

Fail _____

Comments: _____

_____

Instructor: _____

© 1994 W.B. Saunders Company. *Rambo's Nursing Skills for Clinical Practice,* fourth edition
All rights reserved.

PERFORMANCE CHECKLIST

Skill 7-7   Perineal care for the female

Student: _____

Date: _____

		Satisfactory	Unsatisfactory
1.	Wash hands, gather equipment, check the order, identify the patient, provide privacy and explain the procedure.	❑	❑
2.	Raise the bed and position the patient.	❑	❑
3.	Drape the patient.	❑	❑
4.	Don gloves and remove the sanitary pad.	❑	❑
5.	Place bedpan under patient.	❑	❑
6.	Pour or squirt warm water over the perineum.	❑	❑
7.	With moistened cotton balls, cleanse the perineum stroking from the front to the back one time for each cotton ball.	❑	❑
8.	Dry the area with cotton balls or tissues, stroking from front to back.	❑	❑
9.	Remove the bedpan; apply a clean pad.	❑	❑
10.	Discard soiled supplies in secured plastic bag.	❑	❑
11.	Make patient comfortable, lower bed.	❑	❑
12.	Remove and clean equipment and return to storage area.	❑	❑
13.	Document the procedure.	❑	❑

Pass _____

Fail _____

Comments: _____

_____

Instructor: _____

© 1994 W.B. Saunders Company. *Rambo's Nursing Skills for Clinical Practice,* fourth edition
All rights reserved.

PERFORMANCE CHECKLIST

Skill 7-8   Grooming the hair

Student: _____

Date: _____

	Satisfactory	**Unsatisfactory**
1. Wash your hands, identify the patient, gather the equipment, and explain the procedure.	❏	❏
2. Drape the patient's shoulders or cover the pillow.	❏	❏
3. Part the hair in the middle and separate into three sections per side.	❏	❏
4. Brush one section at a time.	❏	❏
5. Comb each section of hair.	❏	❏
6. Arrange hair neatly.	❏	❏
7. Remove the towel or drape.	❏	❏
8. Tidy the area.	❏	❏

Pass _____

Fail _____

Comments: _____

_____

Instructor: _____

© 1994 W.B. Saunders Company. *Rambo's Nursing Skills for Clinical Practice,* fourth edition
All rights reserved.

PERFORMANCE CHECKLIST

Skill 7-9   Braiding the hair

Student: _____

Date: _____

	Satisfactory	Unsatisfactory
1. Wash your hands, identify the patient, and explain the procedure.	❑	❑
2. Divide the freshly brushed and combed hair into three sections on each side.	❑	❑
3. Braid the hair.	❑	❑
4. Secure the braid.	❑	❑
5. Make patient comfortable; tidy the area.	❑	❑

Pass _____

Fail _____

Comments: _____

_____

Instructor: _____

© 1994 W.B. Saunders Company. *Rambo's Nursing Skills for Clinical Practice,* fourth edition
All rights reserved.

PERFORMANCE CHECKLIST

Skill 7-10   Shampooing the hair

Student: _____

Date: _____

	Satisfactory	Unsatisfactory
1. Check the order, assemble the equipment, identify the patient, explain the procedure, raise the bed and provide privacy.	❑	❑
2. Protect the bed linen at the top of the bed.	❑	❑
3. Position the patient at the side of the bed.	❑	❑
4. Drape the patient.	❑	❑
5. Slip shampoo tray under patient's head.	❑	❑
6. Position drainage receptacle beneath shampoo tray spout.	❑	❑
7. Fill pitcher with warm water.	❑	❑
8. Moisten the hair before applying shampoo.	❑	❑
9. Apply shampoo and work into hair from front to back massaging scalp firmly.	❑	❑
10. Rinse the hair thoroughly.	❑	❑
11. Reapply shampoo as in step 9.	❑	❑
12. Rinse until hair strand produces squeaky sound when rubbed between fingers.	❑	❑
13. Towel dry the hair, face, and neck thoroughly.	❑	❑
14. Brush the hair and comb out tangles.	❑	❑
15. Dry hair with hair dryer if desired.	❑	❑
16. Remove equipment and soiled towels.	❑	❑
17. Make patient comfortable.	❑	❑
18. Lower the bed, tidy the area.	❑	❑
19. Document the procedure.	❑	❑

FOR STRETCHER SHAMPOO

	Satisfactory	Unsatisfactory
1. Bring stretcher alongside bed and transfer patient to stretcher.	❑	❑
2. Transport patient to shampoo area.	❑	❑
3. Place stretcher with patient's head over sink and lock the wheels.	❑	❑
4. Place a towel around shoulders and neck.	❑	❑

© 1994 W.B. Saunders Company. *Rambo's Nursing Skills for Clinical Practice,* fourth edition
All rights reserved.

5. Adjust water to warm flow. ❑ ❑

6. With sprayer device, wet hair. ❑ ❑

7. Shampoo as in steps 9 through 15 above. ❑ ❑

8. Return patient to room, positioning stretcher alongside the bed. ❑ ❑

9. Transfer the patient to the bed; cover and make comfortable. ❑ ❑

10. Lower the bed, raise the siderails, replace call bell. ❑ ❑

11. Document the procedure. ❑ ❑

Pass _____

Fail _____

Comments: _____

_____

Instructor: _____

© 1994 W.B. Saunders Company. *Rambo's Nursing Skills for Clinical Practice,* fourth edition
All rights reserved.

PERFORMANCE CHECKLIST

Skill 7-11 Shaving the male patient

Student: _____

Date: _____

	Satisfactory	Unsatisfactory
1. Wash your hands, gather the equipment, identify the patient, and explain the procedure.	❏	❏
2. Position in seated or Fowler's position.	❏	❏
3. Drape the chest and shoulders.	❏	❏
FOR ELECTRIC RAZOR		
4. Apply pre-shave lotion.	❏	❏
5. Hold skin taut and shave with short strokes in direction of hair growth.	❏	❏
FOR SAFETY RAZOR		
6. Soften beard with warm, moist towel.	❏	❏
7. Apply shaving cream.	❏	❏
8. With skin taut, use short strokes and shave in the direction of hair growth without cutting skin.	❏	❏
9. Rinse face with wet washcloth and pat dry.	❏	❏
10. Apply aftershave lotion.	❏	❏
11. Make patient comfortable and tidy area.	❏	❏
12. Clean equipment and replace in storage area.	❏	❏
13. Document procedure.	❏	❏

Pass _____

Fail _____

Comments: _____

_____

Instructor: _____

© 1994 W.B. Saunders Company. *Rambo's Nursing Skills for Clinical Practice,* fourth edition
All rights reserved.

Suggested Clinical Activities

1. Practice the bed bath procedure at home on a family member or friend until you are comfortable and efficient with the procedure.

2. Practice shaving the face of a male family member or friend to decrease initial anxiety and awkwardness when performing the procedure in the health care agency.

3. Accompany another nurse when she gives hygiene care to an unconscious patient. Pay particular attention to technique of giving safe mouth care.

4. When observing hygiene care being given by other nurses, notice how the patient's privacy is protected or invaded. Discuss this issue in clinical conference.

5. Practice braiding long hair on a friend of classmate until you are comfortable with the technique.

6. Assist another nurse in giving a bed shampoo in order to become more familiar and comfortable with this task.

© 1994 W.B. Saunders Company. *Rambo's Nursing Skills for Clinical Practice,* fourth edition
All rights reserved.

Chapter 8

The Environment and Environmental Safety

LEARNING ACTIVITIES

I. Fill in the blanks with the correct words.

1. Environment consists of all things that affect the _____ or _____ of a person.

2. On of the most common places falls occur in the hospital is when the patient is attempting to go to the

   _____.

3. In order to decrease odors within the patient's environment, all used dressings, catheters and other removed tubes

   should be contained in a closed impermeable bag or _____ from the room.

4. The patient's environment should be straightened at least _____.

5. The acronym RACE stands for:

   R _____

   A _____

   C _____

   E_____

6. One reason geriatric patients are more at risk for injury is that they often have decreased _____.

7. The nurse performs a key role in _____ safety when she carefully inspects equipment before
   plugging it in for use.

© 1994 W.B. Saunders Company. *Rambo's Nursing Skills for Clinical Practice,* fourth edition
All rights reserved.

8. List three methods of providing a patient with additional warmth (a doctor's order is required for some):

    a. _____

    b. _____

    c. _____

9. List the three types of patients who require *very special care* if external heat is applied because they could be burned easily:

    a. _____

    b. _____

    c. _____

10. While making a bed, the nurse utilizes principles of asepsis and _____ the bed to proper working

    _____.

11. Hospital beds are made so that the linens stay as "tucked" as possible. The most common method of doing this is to

    _____ the corners.

12. Linens are never "fanned" during bedmaking as this tends to cause air currents that spread

    _____.

13. The purpose of a draw sheet is to _____.

14. A draw sheet may be used as a lift sheet and is useful in _____ the person in bed.

15. When making a postoperative or "surgical" bed, the bed itself should be left in _____ position

    with the covers _____.

COMPLETE THE FOLLOWING STATEMENTS

16. A good light is bright enough to avoid straining the eyes in order to see, but it should be diffused or without

    _____.

17. Why is a night-light desirable in a hospital room? _____

© 1994 W.B. Saunders Company. *Rambo's Nursing Skills for Clinical Practice,* fourth edition
All rights reserved.

18. The colors in a room *(can) (cannot)* affect a person who is not colorblind.

19. Most patient rooms in hospitals have *(subdued pastel colors) (bright stimulating colors)*.

20. List three common sources of hospital noise.

    a. _____

    b. _____

    c. _____

21. How do you think *you* can best reduce undesirable noise in your hospital?

    a. _____

    b. _____

22. List two ways in which the patient may be a source of unpleasant odors.

    a. _____

    b. _____

23. List two ways in which the worker may be a source of unpleasant odors.

    a. _____

    b. _____

24. List two ways in which the room or hospital might be a source of odors.

    a. _____

    b. _____

25. Lsit three ways in which you can provide privacy for your patient.

    a. _____

    b. _____

    c. _____

© 1994 W.B. Saunders Company. *Rambo's Nursing Skills for Clinical Practice,* fourth edition
All rights reserved.

26. Falls cause many accidents in and out of hospitals. List five ways in which you might prevent falls.

a. _____

b. _____

c. _____

d. _____

e. _____

II. Take the post-test included at the end of the chapter in the text.

© 1994 W.B. Saunders Company. *Rambo's Nursing Skills for Clinical Practice,* fourth edition
All rights reserved.

PERFORMANCE CHECKLIST

Skill 8-1   Promoting patient safety during a fire

Student: _____

Date: _____

	Satisfactory	Unsatisfactory
1. States first step is to evacuate persons in immediate fire area to a safe place.	❏	❏
2. States then would activate fire alarm and indicates location.	❏	❏
3. States would close all doors and windows in vicinity of fire and turn off oxygen in the room.	❏	❏
4. Identifies correct type of extinguisher to be used on the fire and knows its location.	❏	❏
5. Describes proper procedure for using the fire extinguisher.	❏	❏
6. States protocol for documentation of a fire.	❏	❏

Pass _____

Fail _____

Comments: _____

_____

Instructor: _____

© 1994 W.B. Saunders Company. *Rambo's Nursing Skills for Clinical Practice,* fourth edition
All rights reserved.

PERFORMANCE CHECKLIST

Skill 8-2 Making an unoccupied bed

Student: _____

Date: _____

		Satisfactory	Unsatisfactory
1.	Carries out Standard Steps A, B, C, D, and E as need indicates.	❏	❏
2.	Arranges linens in order they will be used before beginning.	❏	❏
3.	Assists patient out of the bed.	❏	❏
4.	Raises bed to correct working height.	❏	❏
5.	Loosens linens, removes spread and/or blanket and folds them for reuse.	❏	❏
6.	Removes the sheets and pillowcases and places them in laundry hamper or bag.	❏	❏
7.	Moves mattress to head of the bed.	❏	❏
8.	Makes bed on one side, mitering corners of sheet and bed covers.	❏	❏
9.	Positions drawsheet correctly if used.	❏	❏
10.	Makes other side of the bed, mitering corners.	❏	❏
11.	Bed is tight and smooth with a cuff at the top of the covers.	❏	❏
12.	Provides a toe pleat if needed.	❏	❏
13.	Applies pillowcases without contaminating them.	❏	❏
14.	Lowers and locks bed, raises far top side rail, attaches call light and places personal articles within reach.	❏	❏
15.	Removes soiled linens without contaminating uniform.	❏	❏
16.	Completes bedmaking within allotted time of _____ minutes.	❏	❏
17.	Carries out Standard Steps X, Y, and Z.	❏	❏

Pass _____

Fail _____

Comments: _____

_____

Instructor: _____

© 1994 W.B. Saunders Company. *Rambo's Nursing Skills for Clinical Practice,* fourth edition
All rights reserved.

PERFORMANCE CHECKLIST

Skill 8-3 Making an occupied bed

Student: _____

Date: _____

	Satisfactory	**Unsatisfactory**
1. Carries out Standard Steps A, B, C, D, and E as need indicates.	❑	❑
2. Raises the bed to working height and raises far side rail before turning the patient.	❑	❑
3. Loosens top covers and removes spread and/or blanket, folds and places them over a chair for reuse if unsoiled.	❑	❑
4. Places bath blanket over the patient and removes the top sheet.	❑	❑
5. Assists patient to a side-lying position on the far side of the bed.	❑	❑
6. Loosens bottom linens and rolls each piece of linen close to the patient.	❑	❑
7. Makes near side of the bed with the bottom linens, mitering the corner at the top of the mattress.	❑	❑
8. Positions drawsheet correctly if used.	❑	❑
9. Raises the siderail before going to other side of the bed.	❑	❑
10. Assists person to move to the other side of the bed.	❑	❑
11. Lowers siderail and loosens bottom linens and removes them; places soiled linens in hamper or bag.	❑	❑
12. Tightens, smooths, and tucks bottom linens in on this side of the bed, mitering the top corner.	❑	❑
13. Positions patient in center of bed in supine position, places top sheet, removes bath blanket, and places spread.	❑	❑
14. Smooths top linens, tucks in and miters the bottom corners, and forms top cuff.	❑	❑
15. Makes room for toes.	❑	❑
16. Changes pillowcases without contaminating them and replaces pillows.	❑	❑
17. Lowers the bed to lowest position, raises siderail, attaches the call light, and places personal items within reach.	❑	❑
18. Removes the soiled linens without contaminating uniform.	❑	❑
19. Completes bedmaking within allotted time of _____ minutes.	❑	❑
20. Carries out Standard Steps X, Y, and Z.	❑	❑

© 1994 W.B. Saunders Company. *Rambo's Nursing Skills for Clinical Practice,* fourth edition
All rights reserved.

Pass _____

Fail _____

Comments: _____

_____

Instructor: _____

© 1994 W.B. Saunders Company. *Rambo's Nursing Skills for Clinical Practice,* fourth edition
All rights reserved.

PERFORMANCE CHECKLIST

Skill 8-4   Preparing the postoperative unit

Student: _____

Date: _____

	Satisfactory	Unsatisfactory
1. Makes an unoccupied bed.	❑	❑
2. Prepares surgical or anesthetic bed by fan folding the covers to the side or bottom.	❑	❑
3. Leaves bed ready to receive patient from stretcher.	❑	❑
4. Places underpads at correct locations.	❑	❑
5. Prepares room for stretcher transfer or patient.	❑	❑
6. Places I. V. pole at head of bed.	❑	❑
7. Places emesis basin and tissues by bed.	❑	❑
8. Removes soiled linens and places clean towels in room.	❑	❑

Pass _____

Fail _____

Comments: _____

_____

Instructor: _____

© 1994 W.B. Saunders Company. *Rambo's Nursing Skills for Clinical Practice,* fourth edition
All rights reserved.

Suggested Clinical Activities

1. During a clinical day, determine if there is adequate provision for a physically comfortable environment. Consider temperature, lighting, ventilation, and humidity.

2. When assigned to a clinical unit, find the fire alarm locations, the fire extinguishers, and study the fire evacuation plan.

3. Practice at least 2 different fire carrys with your friends or a classmate.

4. Practice hospital bedmaking at home until you can complete the process in 3–5 minutes.

© 1994 W.B. Saunders Company. *Rambo's Nursing Skills for Clinical Practice,* fourth edition
All rights reserved.

Chapter 9

Safety Devices and Techniques (Restraints)

LEARNING ACTIVITIES

I. Fill in the blanks with the correct word or phrase.

1. Give three reasons why a safety device (restraint) might be employed.

    a. _____

    b. _____

    c. _____

2. Five adverse effects of the long-term use of devices that restrict movement include

    a. _____

    b. _____

    c. _____

    d. _____

    e. _____

3. Psychological effects of immobilization by safety devices often include _____ and

    _____.

4. An immobilization device is never solely used to _____

    _____.

5. When an immobilization device is used, the nurse must document the _____ requiring the use of the immobilizing device.

6. Four nursing actions to promote patient safety include:

   a. _____

   b. _____

   c. _____

   d. _____

7. One action that helps prevent patient falls is to place personal items close at hand so that the patient does not have

   to _____.

8. To prevent falls in the home, _____ should be installed at the toilet, in the tub and shower.

9. To prevent falls when transferring from or to the wheelchair, be certain _____

   _____.

10. Safety devices must _____ the patient or be necessary for the continuation of _____

    _____.

11. Rather than securing a patient's arms when tubes are in danger of being pulled out, _____ might be tried.

12. If an immobilization device is applied in an emergency situation to protect the patient, the physician must sign

    an order within _____ hours.

13. Immobilization devices are never used to _____ the patient.

14. Whenever a security or immobilization device is applied, the nurse must frequently check _____

    and _____ function.

15. If a patient has an extremity immobilized, his position must be changed every _____ and the joints

    must be _____.

16. Often the decision that the security device is no longer necessary is up to the _____.

17. To secure a patient in a wheelchair, either a _____ or a _____ can be
    used.

© 1994 W.B. Saunders Company. *Rambo's Nursing Skills for Clinical Practice,* fourth edition
All rights reserved.

18. The ties of a security device used for a bed patient should be tied to _____

19. When a patient is confused, the nurse in her assessment of the cause should check the _____
_____.

20. Before resorting to a security device to protect the patient, the nurse must _____
_____.

II. Take the post-test included at the end of the chapter in the text.

© 1994 W.B. Saunders Company. *Rambo's Nursing Skills for Clinical Practice,* fourth edition
All rights reserved.

PERFORMANCE CHECKLIST

Skill 9-1   Applying a security/safety belt

Student: _____

Date: _____

	Satisfactory	Unsatisfactory
1. Carries out Standard Steps A, B, C, D, and E as need indicates.	❏	❏
2. Applies security belt correctly.	❏	❏
3. Ties securing knot correctly.	❏	❏
4. Checks patient every 30 minutes.	❏	❏
5. Identifies safety precautions to be used with this device.	❏	❏
6. Includes all pertinent points in documentation for use of this device.	❏	❏
7. Carries out Standard Steps X, Y, and Z.	❏	❏

Pass   _____

Fail   _____

Comments: _____

_____

Instructor: _____

© 1994 W.B. Saunders Company. *Rambo's Nursing Skills for Clinical Practice,* fourth edition
All rights reserved.

PERFORMANCE CHECKLIST

Skill 9-2 Applying a vest security device

Student: _____

Date: _____

	Satisfactory	Unsatisfactory
1. Carries out Standard Steps A, B, C, D, and E as need indicates.	❏	❏
2. Applies security vest correctly.	❏	❏
3. Ties securing knot correctly.	❏	❏
4. Checks patient every 30 minutes.	❏	❏
5. Identifies safety precautions to be used with this device.	❏	❏
6. Includes all pertinent points in documentation for use of this device.	❏	❏
7. Carries out Standard Steps X, Y, and Z.	❏	❏

Pass _____

Fail _____

Comments: _____

_____

Instructor: _____

© 1994 W.B. Saunders Company. *Rambo's Nursing Skills for Clinical Practice,* fourth edition
All rights reserved.

PERFORMANCE CHECKLIST

Skill 9-4   Applying an extremity immobilizer

Student: _____

Date: _____

	Satisfactory	Unsatisfactory
1. Carries out Standard Steps A, B, C, D, and E as need indicates.	❏	❏
2. Applies immobilizer correctly; uses assistant to help as needed.	❏	❏
3. Ties securing knot correctly and to right part of bed.	❏	❏
4. Checks patient every 30 minutes.	❏	❏
5. Removes immobilizer from each extremity, one at a time, every two hours and exercises limb.	❏	❏
6. Identifies safety precautions to be used with this device.	❏	❏
7. Includes all pertinent points in documentation for use of this device.	❏	❏
8. Carries out Standard Steps X, Y, and Z.	❏	❏

Pass _____

Fail _____

Comments: _____

_____

Instructor: _____

© 1994 W.B. Saunders Company. *Rambo's Nursing Skills for Clinical Practice,* fourth edition
All rights reserved.

Suggested Clinical Activities

1. If security and immobilization devices are available in the skill lab, work with a peer and experience wearing such a device.

2. With a classmate, practice tying the ties of a security device to the bed properly.

3. When assigned to a patient who is placed in a security or immobilization device, think creatively to see if there is another solution or way to solve the underlying problem.

© 1994 W.B. Saunders Company. *Rambo's Nursing Skills for Clinical Practice,* fourth edition
All rights reserved.

Chapter 10

Infection Control

LEARNING ACTIVITIES

I. Fill in the blanks with the appropriate word or phrase.

1. Two purposes of using isolation procedures are:

    a. _____

    b. _____

2. Three methods of barrier technique are:

    a. _____

    b. _____

    c. _____

3. The most important method of preventing the spread of microorganisms is _____

    _____ .

4. A nosocomial infection is one that is _____ .

5. Give three examples of nosocomial infections:

    a. _____

    b. _____

    c. _____

6. For a gown to act as a sufficient barrier, it must be _____ .

7. When cleaning up the bed and the patient when incontinence has occurred, the nurse should wear gloves and

    _____ .

All rights reserved.

8. When putting on personal protective equipment to enter an isolation room, when all equipment is used, it should be

    donned in this order: _____.

9. Whenever gloves are worn, the hands are washed _____

    _____.

10. Sharps are disposed of in _____.

11. Four ways to help prevent nosocomial infections are:

    a. _____

    b. _____

    c. _____

    d. _____

12. Isolation precautions are used to control or eliminate the _____ in the chain of infection, control or
    eliminate the _____, interrupt _____, and to _____ susceptible pa-
    tients, staff, and visitors.

13. When removing soiled linens or trash from an isolation unit, the nurse must _____

    _____.

14. Specimens taken from a patient in an isolation unit must be _____

    _____.

15. Visitors to an isolation unit must be reminded that no articles should be _____

    _____.

16. Universal precautions are used for _____.

17. Respiratory isolation would be an example of _____ isolation.

18. When working with a patient under enteric precautions, the nurse must use gloves for _____

    _____.

© 1994 W.B. Saunders Company. *Rambo's Nursing Skills for Clinical Practice,* fourth edition
All rights reserved.

19. A serious disease requiring isolation that is steadily increasing in incidence in the United States is _____

    _____.

20. Protective isolation is for the purpose of _____

    _____.

II. *True or False. Circle the "T" if the statement is true or "F" if the statement is false.*

T F   1. All articles used for or by the patient in an isolation unit are considered contaminated.
T F   2. It is necessary to wear a gown when giving a bedpan.
T F   3. Unused articles and linens are not to be removed from an isolation unit and placed with other articles and linens for use by other patients.
T F   4. Microorganisms inflict damage to the patient through their ability to produce certain toxins.
T F   5. Linens removed from an isolation unit must be placed in an additional bag as well as the original bag in which they are placed.
T F   6. A patient in a respiratory isolation unit should not be given a backrub with the bare hands.
T F   7. The faucet in the isolation bathroom is considered clean and suitable to turn on and off without protection.
T F   8. Isolation technique dictates that a mask is always worn.
T F   9. Food trays may be served to the patient in isolation in regular fashion since all trays are sterilized in the dishwasher.
T F 10. TPR may be taken without a gown so long as the uniform does not touch anything in all types of isolation rooms.

III. *Take the post-test included at the end of the chapter in the text.*

© 1994 W.B. Saunders Company. *Rambo's Nursing Skills for Clinical Practice,* fourth edition
All rights reserved.

PERFORMANCE CHECKLIST

Skill 10-1   Donning personal protective equipment: Gown and mask

Student: _____

Date: _____

	Satisfactory	Unsatisfactory
1. Obtains clean gown and unfolds it.	❏	❏
2. Places arms into the sleeves, works arms through sleeves, and adjusts at shoulders.	❏	❏
3. Ties neck tapes, closes gown at the back and ties waist tie.	❏	❏
4. Obtains a mask from the container.	❏	❏
5. Places the outside of the mask over the nose and mouth.	❏	❏
6. Positions the rubber band or ties the ties over the ears and around the neck.	❏	❏
7. Adjusts the nose band so that mask will not slip.	❏	❏

Pass _____

Fail _____

Comments: _____

_____

Instructor: _____

© 1994 W.B. Saunders Company. *Rambo's Nursing Skills for Clinical Practice,* fourth edition
All rights reserved.

PERFORMANCE CHECKLIST

Skill 10-2   Removing gloves and isolation gown

Date:_____

Student: _____

	Satisfactory	Unsatisfactory
1. Unties the waist tie.	❏	❏
2. Removes one glove without contaminating own skin.	❏	❏
3. Holds removed glove in other gloved hand; removes other glove without contaminating own skin.	❏	❏
4. Disposes of gloves in trash receptacle.	❏	❏
5. Slides off gown without touching the outside of it.	❏	❏
6. Folds or rolls gown inside out and places in trash receptacle or linen hamper.	❏	❏
7. Washes hands.	❏	❏

Pass _____

Fail _____

Comments: _____

_____

Instructor: _____

© 1994 W.B. Saunders Company. *Rambo's Nursing Skills for Clinical Practice,* fourth edition
All rights reserved.

PERFORMANCE CHECKLIST

Skill 10-3   Double bagging technique

Date: _____

Student: _____

	Satisfactory	**Unsatisfactory**
1. Seals the first impervious bag while inside the room.	❏	❏
2. Places sealed bag inside outer bag held by nurse outside of room without contaminating the outside or edges of the outer bag.	❏	❏

AS OUTSIDE NURSE:

1. Holds outer impervious bag with cuff at top over hands.	❏	❏
2. After inside nurse deposits the inner bag, secures the outer bag without touching the inner bag's top.	❏	❏
3. Disposes of the double bagged material per agency policy.	❏	❏

Pass _____

Fail _____

Comments: _____

_____

Instructor: _____

© 1994 W.B. Saunders Company. *Rambo's Nursing Skills for Clinical Practice,* fourth edition
All rights reserved.

Suggested Clinical Activities

1. Locate on your assigned unit where the items of personal protective equipment are kept.

2. Practice removing gloves without contaminating your hands; have a classmate watch so that mistakes will be caught.

3. Review the correct technique for handwashing.

4. While on the clinical unit, observe other nurses washing their hands; do they comply with the recommended technique?

5. Inspect an isolation cart.

6. Accompany a nurse into an isolation room and help care for the patient.

7. Review the types of isolation used in your assigned health care facility in the procedure manual.

© 1994 W.B. Saunders Company. *Rambo's Nursing Skills for Clinical Practice,* fourth edition
All rights reserved.

Chapter 11

Vital Signs, Height and Weight

LEARNING ACTIVITIES

I. Answer the following questions based on information about body temperature.

1. Why would you take the patient's vital signs at frequent intervals during a period of illness?

   _____

2. What is the normal temperature of a healthy person in degrees Fahrenheit? _____

3. What is the normal temperature in degrees Celsius? _____

4. Above what temperature is a person considered to have a fever? _____

5. Name at least four factors that influence body temperature:

   a. _____

   b. _____

   c. _____

   d. _____

6. List the four most common sites used for taking the body temperature:

   a. _____

   b. _____

   c. _____

   d. _____

7. With a fever of two degrees (F) above normal, how much is the metabolic rate increased?

_____

8. List the three fever classifications:

a. _____

b. _____

c. _____

9. What is the nrmal range for pulse in a health adult? _____

10. In addition to the rate, what characteristics of the pulse should you note and be able to describe? _____

_____

11. List the points on the body where the pulse can be palpated. _____

12. What is the medical term used to describe a pulse of 48? _____

13. What is the medical term used to describe a pulse of 128? _____

14. Name at least six factors that might increase the pulse rate.

a. _____

b. _____

c. _____

d. _____

e. _____

f. _____

15. What are the three types of abnormal pulse that you would report to the nurse or to the physician?

a. _____

b. _____

c. _____

© 1994 W.B. Saunders Company. *Rambo's Nursing Skills for Clinical Practice,* fourth edition
All rights reserved.

16. The normal range of respirations for a healthy adult is _____.

17. The respiratory center of the brain is more sensitive to changes in the _____ levels in the blood.

18. What is the ratio most often found between the number of respirations and the number of pulse beats? _____

19. The normal pattern of breathing is described as _____.

20. Any type of noisy breathing should be regarded as _____.

21. What is the term used to describe difficult and labored breathing? _____.

22. What is the name of the breathing pattern that occurs in cycles with rapid, difficult breathing following by a period of no breathing? _____.

II. Answer the questions and fill in the blanks.

1. The normal blood pressure in healthy young adults is _____.

2. Systolic pressure refers to the (highest) (lowest) pressure caused by the contraction of the ventricules. _____.

3. Which pressure reading is written below the line in BP? _____.

4. How do you determine pulse pressure, the force we can feel when taking the pulse? _____ _____.

5. BP measurements above what level indicate hypertension? _____.

6. Name at least five factors that cause an elevation in the blood pressure.

   a. _____

   b. _____

   c. _____

© 1994 W.B. Saunders Company. *Rambo's Nursing Skills for Clinical Practice,* fourth edition
All rights reserved.

d. _____

e. _____

7. Low blood pressures are dangerous when they occur with symptoms of _____.

III. Fill in the blanks or answer the questions.

1. Name two types of manometers most commonly used by nurses to take blood pressures.

a. _____

b. _____

2. The blood pressure is usually measured over an artery at what site? _____

3. Describe the sound that indicates the systolic pressure. _____

4. Describe the sounds that are associated with the diastolic pressure. _____

5. To avoid making errors in reading the pressure, where should the manometer gauge be located?
   _____

6. Why would you palpate the brachial or radial artery before taking the blood pressure? _____
   _____

IV. Answer the following questions based on information about height:

1. Adults are usually measured in a _____ position.

2. _____ is used to measure infants and children under three years.

3. _____ and _____ are units commonly used to measure height.

V. List three physical factors that can affect a person's actual height:

a. _____, b. _____, and c. _____.

© 1994 W.B. Saunders Company. *Rambo's Nursing Skills for Clinical Practice,* fourth edition
All rights reserved.

Answer the following questions based on information about weight.

4. List three types of scales:

   a. _____

   b. _____

   c. _____

5. A person who is able to stand is weighed on a _____ scale.

6. A person who cannot stand may be weighed on a _____ scale, or a _____ scale.

7. One purpose of daily weights is _____.

8. List two external factors that affect weight measurement:

   a. _____

   and

   b. _____

VI. Take the post-test included at the end of the chapter in the text.

© 1994 W.B. Saunders Company. *Rambo's Nursing Skills for Clinical Practice,* fourth edition
All rights reserved.

PERFORMANCE CHECKLIST

Skill 11-1   Measuring the temperature with a glass thermometer

Student: _____

Date: _____

	Satisfactory	Unsatisfactory
FOR ORAL TEMPERATURE		
1. Carries out Standard Steps A, B, C, D, and E as need indicates.	❑	❑
2. Cleans and ascertains that thermometer mercury is below 96°F.	❑	❑
3. Checks when patient last had something to eat or drink.	❑	❑
4. Place thermometer under the tongue and asks patient to close lips.	❑	❑
5. Leaves thermometer in mouth for at least three minutes.	❑	❑
6. Removes and wipes thermometer from top to bulb.	❑	❑
7. Reads thermometer measurement correctly.	❑	❑
8. Records temperature measurement accurately.	❑	❑
9. Cleans and replaces thermometer.	❑	❑
10. Carries out Standard Steps X, Y, and Z.	❑	❑

Pass _____

Fail _____

Comments: _____

_____

Instructor: _____

© 1994 W.B. Saunders Company. *Rambo's Nursing Skills for Clinical Practice,* fourth edition
All rights reserved.

PERFORMANCE CHECKLIST

Skill 11-2   Measuring the temperature with an electronic thermometer

Student: _____

Date: _____

	Satisfactory	Unsatisfactory
1. Carries out Standard Steps A, B, C, D, and E as need indicates.	❏	❏
2. Places probe cover over probe.	❏	❏
3. Places thermometer probe in patient's mouth with thermometer turned on.	❏	❏
4. Waits until machine indicates temperature reading is complete.	❏	❏
5. Disposes of probe cover.	❏	❏
6. Records temperature.	❏	❏
7. Turns off unit by returning probe to base.	❏	❏
8. Carries out Standard Steps X, Y, and Z.	❏	❏

Pass _____

Fail _____

Comments: _____

_____

Instructor: _____

© 1994 W.B. Saunders Company. *Rambo's Nursing Skills for Clinical Practice,* fourth edition
All rights reserved.

PERFORMANCE CHECKLIST

Skill 11-3   Measuring the temperature with a tympanic thermometer

Student: _____

Date: _____

	Satisfactory	**Unsatisfactory**
1. Carries out Standard Steps A, B, C, D, and E as need indicates.	❏	❏
2. Readies tympanic thermometer unit and places probe cover over the probe.	❏	❏
3. Inspects ear canal and places probe in auditory canal.	❏	❏
4. Steadies tympanic thermometer unit.	❏	❏
5. Reads tympanic temperature accurately and removes probe from ear.	❏	❏
6. Discards probe cover.	❏	❏
7. Returns probe to base tympanic thermometer unit.	❏	❏
8. Records tympanic temperature accurately.	❏	❏
9. Carries out Standard Steps X, Y, and Z.	❏	❏

Pass _____

Fail _____

Comments: _____

_____

Instructor: _____

© 1994 W.B. Saunders Company. *Rambo's Nursing Skills for Clinical Practice,* fourth edition
All rights reserved.

PERFORMANCE CHECKLIST

Skill 11-4   Measuring a radial pulse

Student: _____

Date: _____

	Satisfactory	Unsatisfactory
1. Carries out Standard Steps A, B, C, D, and E as need indicates.	❑	❑
2. Locates radial pulse using pads of fingers.	❑	❑
3. Counts radial pulse accurately for 30 seconds.	❑	❑
4. Records radial pulse rate accurately.	❑	❑
5. Reports any abnormalities.	❑	❑
6. Carries out Standard Steps X, Y, and Z.	❑	❑

Pass _____

Fail _____

Comments: _____

_____

Instructor: _____

© 1994 W.B. Saunders Company. *Rambo's Nursing Skills for Clinical Practice,* fourth edition
All rights reserved.

PERFORMANCE CHECKLIST

Skill 11-6   Measuring an apical pulse

Student: _____

Date: _____

	Satisfactory	Unsatisfactory
1. Carries out Standard Steps A, B, C, D, and E as need indicates.	❑	❑
2. Exposes chest and correctly locates apex of heart area.	❑	❑
3. Listens and counts apical pulse rate accurately for 60 seconds.	❑	❑
4. Records the apical pulse rate accurately.	❑	❑
5. Carries out Standard Steps X, Y, and Z.	❑	❑

Pass _____

Fail _____

Comments: _____

_____

Instructor: _____

© 1994 W.B. Saunders Company. *Rambo's Nursing Skills for Clinical Practice,* fourth edition
All rights reserved.

PERFORMANCE CHECKLIST

Skill 11-5   Measuring an apical-radial pulse rate

Student: _____

Date: _____

	Satisfactory	**Unsatisfactory**
1. Carries out Standard Steps A, B, C, D, and E as need indicates.	❏	❏
2. Positions watch where both nurses can see it.	❏	❏
3. Signals when to begin counting.	❏	❏
4. Auscultates and counts apical pulse for one full minute while partner palpates and counts radial pulse.	❏	❏
5. States "stop" on the 60 second count.	❏	❏
6. Identifies pulse differences (deficit) between the apical and radial pulse rate.	❏	❏
7. Records the apical pulse rate and any pulse deficit accurately.	❏	❏
8. Carries out Standard Steps X, Y, and Z.	❏	❏

Pass _____

Fail _____

Comments: _____

_____

Instructor: _____

© 1994 W.B. Saunders Company. *Rambo's Nursing Skills for Clinical Practice,* fourth edition
All rights reserved.

PERFORMANCE CHECKLIST

Skill 11-7   Measuring respirations

Student: _____

Date: _____

	Satisfactory	**Unsatisfactory**
1. Carries out Standard Steps A, B, C, D, and E as need indicates.	❏	❏
2. Counts the respirations accurately noting rate, depth, and character.	❏	❏
3. Records the respiratory rate accurately.	❏	❏
4. Carries out Standard Steps X, Y, and Z.	❏	❏

Pass _____

Fail _____

Comments: _____

_____

Instructor: _____

© 1994 W.B. Saunders Company. *Rambo's Nursing Skills for Clinical Practice,* fourth edition
All rights reserved.

PERFORMANCE CHECKLIST

Skill 11-8   Measuring blood pressure

Student: _____

Date: _____

	Satisfactory	Unsatisfactory
1. Carries out Standard Steps A, B, C, D, and E as need indicates.	❑	❑
2. Positions patient and allows to rest for five minutes before taking BP.	❑	❑
3. Applies correct size cuff to arm correctly.	❑	❑
4. Palpates brachial pulse; inflates cuff until brachial pulse disappears; deflates cuff.	❑	❑
5. Places stethoscope diaphragm over brachial pulse and inflates cuff to a point 30 mm Hg above point where pulse disappears.	❑	❑
6. Slowly deflates cuff while listening for Korotkoff sounds.	❑	❑
7. Identifies accurate systolic and diastolic blood pressure measurement.	❑	❑
8. Records systolic and diastolic blood pressure.	❑	❑
9. Repeats procedure if uncertain readings are accurate.	❑	❑
10. Carries out Standard Steps X, Y, and Z.	❑	❑

Pass _____

Fail _____

Comments: _____

_____

Instructor: _____

© 1994 W.B. Saunders Company. *Rambo's Nursing Skills for Clinical Practice,* fourth edition
All rights reserved.

PERFORMANCE CHECKLIST

Skill 11-9 Measuring height

Student: _____

Date: _____

	Satisfactory	Unsatisfactory
1. Carries out Standard Steps A, B, C, D, and E as need indicates.	❏	❏
2. Has patient remove shoes.	❏	❏
3. Assists patient to stand on scale platform and assume correct posture.	❏	❏
4. Adjusts measuring device.	❏	❏
5. Obtains accurate height measurement.	❏	❏
6. Records height measurement accurately.	❏	❏
7. Carries out Standard Steps X, Y, and Z.	❏	❏

Pass _____

Fail _____

Comments: _____

_____

Instructor: _____

© 1994 W.B. Saunders Company. *Rambo's Nursing Skills for Clinical Practice,* fourth edition
All rights reserved.

PERFORMANCE CHECKLIST

Skill 11-10   Measuring weight for an adult

Student: _____

Date: _____

	Satisfactory	Unsatisfactory
1. Carries out Standard Steps A, B, C, D, and E as need indicates.	❏	❏
2. Calibrates or balances the scale.	❏	❏
3. Assists patient to stand on scale platform or positions in appropriate scale.	❏	❏
4. Weighs patient accurately.	❏	❏
5. Records weight accurately.	❏	❏
6. Assists patient off of scale.	❏	❏
7. Carries out Standard Steps X, Y, and Z.	❏	❏

Pass _____

Fail _____

Comments: _____

_____

Instructor: _____

© 1994 W.B. Saunders Company. *Rambo's Nursing Skills for Clinical Practice,* fourth edition.
All rights reserved.

PERFORMANCE CHECKLIST

Skill 11-11   Measuring weight for an infant

Student: _____

Date: _____

	Satisfactory	Unsatisfactory
1. Carries out Standard Steps A, B, C, D, and E as need indicates.	❑	❑
2. Insures warm temperature in room	❑	❑
3. Places shield over weighing surface.	❑	❑
4. Places infant on scale.	❑	❑
5. Weighs infant accurately.	❑	❑
6. Records weight accurately.	❑	❑
7. Removes infant from scale.	❑	❑
8. Carries out Standard Steps X, Y, and Z.	❑	❑

Pass _____

Fail _____

Comments: _____

_____

Instructor: _____

© 1994 W.B. Saunders Company. *Rambo's Nursing Skills for Clinical Practice,* fourth edition
All rights reserved.

Suggested Clinical Activities

1. Practice taking an oral temperature using a glass thermometer. Work with a peer who knows how to read the glass thermometer if you have never used one.

2. If a tympanic thermometer is available in your Skill Lab, practice taking temperatures on several different people.

3. If possible, check out a blood pressure cuff from the Skill Lab and practice taking blood pressure on every one who will let you check the pressure. Initially work with another nurse or a classmate who is comfortable with the procedure. Have a classmate check your measurements on a few people to see if you are accurate. There may be a few points of variance when the blood pressure is not taken at exactly the same time by both people. If you cannot check out a BP cuff, plan time to do this exercise in the lab or clinical setting. Try to use both a portable sphygmomanometer and a standing sphygmomanometer.

4. Work with a classmate and check the respiratory rate on five people. You should both have the same results.

5. Practice taking the radial pulse on ten different people. Have a classmate check the pulse by counting at the same time on a least three people to be certain that you are accurate.

6. Take the apical pulse on five different people. Have a classmate or instructor check your results. You should be within a couple of beats of each other.

7. Using a balance scale, correctly weigh three people.

8. Measure three adults.

Practice charting the following vital signs on the Graphic Chart. Be sure to enter the dates and connect the dots for one temperature reading with the dot for the next temperature reading, and do the same for the pulse and respiration values.

Day	8 A.M.	12 noon	4 P.M.	8 P.M.
1	100.2–88–20 160/88	100.8–92–22	102.4–108–24 156/86	103.2–112–24
2	99.6–96–20 148/88	100.6–200–22	100.8–102–22 134/70	98.8–80–18
3	98–76–20 130/80		98.6–72–18 144/88	
4	96.8–66–16 110/70		98.4–84–18 114/64	

Check your work for accuracy with your instructor or another student.

© 1994 W.B. Saunders Company. *Rambo's Nursing Skills for Clinical Practice,* fourth edition
All rights reserved.

Chapter 12

Assessment and Physical Examination

LEARNING ACTIVITIES

I. Indicate the body location(s) to which the following terms apply:

1. ascites _____

2. auscultation _____

3. bruit _____

4. crackles _____

5. cyanosis _____

6. distention _____

7. erythema _____

8. jaundice _____

9. murmur _____

10. pallor _____

11. sigmoidoscope _____

12. speculum _____

13. tinnitus _____

14. turgor _____

15. wheeze _____

II. Fill in the blank(s) with the appropriate word or phrases.

1. For the nurse, assessment is a _____ process.

2. The staff nurse must be adept at performing quick, _____ assessments.

3. Initial patient assessment includes both physical data and _____ data collection.

4. The most helpful of the assessment techniques nurses use is _____.

5. A type of touch frequently used during assessment is _____.

6. Another valuable assessment tool is the _____ used for _____ of the heart, lungs, and abdomen.

7. The nurse auscultates the abdomen, listening for _____ sounds which indicate that the _____ system is functioning.

8. A method of organizing a total patient assessment given in the chapter is the _____ approach.

9. The acronym utilized for the above type of assessment approach is _____.

10. A neurological examination is a rapid way of determining the condition of the _____.

11. The areas and responses assessed during the neurological examination or "check" are:

    a. _____

    b. _____

    c. _____

    d. _____

12. A physical assessment usually is performed starting at the _____.

13. The physical examination generally includes the following major areas:

    a. _____

    b. _____

    c. _____

    d. _____

    e. _____

    f. _____

    g. _____

14. The lithotomy position is generally used for the _____ exam.

© 1994 W.B. Saunders Company. *Rambo's Nursing Skills for Clinical Practice,* fourth edition
All rights reserved.

15. The knee-chest position is generally used for the _____ or _____ exam.

16. The purpose of draping the patient for the physical examination is to_____

_____.

17. Protecting the patient's modesty and privacy during the physical examination helps him/her to _____ and

be more able to _____.

18. To properly perform a visual acuity with the Snellen eye chart, the chart should be _____ until the test
is started.

19. A decrease in the ability to hear as well through air conduction as through bone conduction is indicative of

_____ hearing loss.

20. When utilizing auscultation to perform physical assessment, the nurse should remember to reduce _____

in the room by asking the patient to _____ and by _____

_____.

III. Fill in the answers to the following questions.

1. When determining the amount of assistance necessary for the patient to perform activities of daily living, the nurse
   would assess the following:

   _____

   _____

   _____

   _____

2. The purposes of the physical and psychosocial assessment include the following:

   a. _____

   b. _____

   c. _____

   d. _____

   e. _____

   f. _____

© 1994 W.B. Saunders Company. *Rambo's Nursing Skills for Clinical Practice,* fourth edition
All rights reserved.

3. Major assessment areas within the basic needs approach to physical and psychosocial assessment are:

a. _____

b. _____

c. _____

d. _____

e. _____

f.

g. _____

IV. Take the post-test included at the end of the chapter in the text.

© 1994 W.B. Saunders Company. *Rambo's Nursing Skills for Clinical Practice,* fourth edition
All rights reserved.

PERFORMANCE CHECKLIST

Skill 12-1 Assisting with a medical examination

Student: _____

Date: _____

	Satisfactory	Unsatisfactory
1. Carries out Standard Steps A, B, C, D, and E as need indicates.	❑	❑
2. Takes the following physical measurements and records them on the patient record:		
a. Temperature, pulse and respiration.	❑	❑
b. Blood pressure.	❑	❑
c. Height and weight.	❑	❑
3. Prepares the patient for the examination:		
a. Has patient void and save specimen.	❑	❑
b. Has patient undress and put on gown.	❑	❑
c. Positions and drapes patient on examining table.	❑	❑
4. Assists the examiner during the examination by handing appropriate equipment and supplies as needed.	❑	❑
5. Assists the patient during the examination, giving reassurance and comfort.	❑	❑
6. Changes the patient's position and re-drapes as needed for various parts of the examination.	❑	❑
7. Carries out orders for additional tests or specimens.	❑	❑
8. Carries out Standard Steps X, Y, and Z.	❑	❑

Pass _____

Fail _____

Comments: _____

_____

Instructor: _____

© 1994 W.B. Saunders Company. *Rambo's Nursing Skills for Clinical Practice,* fourth edition
All rights reserved.

PERFORMANCE CHECKLIST

Skill 12-2   Nursing assessment of heart sounds and lung sounds

Student: _____

Date: _____

	Satisfactory	Unsatisfactory
1. Carries out Standard Steps A, B, C, D, and E as need indicates.	❏	❏
2. Positions patient in sitting position or with head of the bed elevated.	❏	❏
3. Listens over bare skin.	❏	❏
4. Eliminates room noise.	❏	❏
5. Auscultates using diaphragm of the stethoscope in all appropriate locations for lung sounds.	❏	❏
6. Auscultates using both diaphragm and bell of the stethoscope for heart sounds in all appropriate locations.	❏	❏
7. Replaces gown or drape.	❏	❏
8. Carries out Standard Steps X, Y, and Z.	❏	❏

Pass _____

Fail _____

Comments: _____

_____

Instructor: _____

© 1994 W.B. Saunders Company. *Rambo's Nursing Skills for Clinical Practice,* fourth edition
All rights reserved.

PERFORMANCE CHECKLIST

Skill 12-3   Neurological check

Student: _____

Date: _____

	Satisfactory	Unsatisfactory
1. Carries out Standard Steps A, B, C, D, and E as need indicates.	❑	❑
2. Asks appropriate questions to determine mental orientation and cognition.	❑	❑
3. Examines pupils for size with room lights subdued; tests pupil constriction in each eye separately.	❑	❑
4. Tests patient's ability to follow a finger to the cardinal points.	❑	❑
5. Tests motor reflexes and ability to follow commands by asking patient to perform certain maneuvers with the extremities.	❑	❑
6. Tests extremity muscle strength by having patient push against hands with the feet and by grasping fingers in each hand.	❑	❑
7. For comatose patient: checks response to a stimulus appropriately.	❑	❑
8. Carries out Standard Steps X, Y, and Z.	❑	❑

Pass _____

Fail _____

Comments: _____

_____

Instructor: _____

© 1994 W.B. Saunders Company. *Rambo's Nursing Skills for Clinical Practice,* fourth edition
All rights reserved.

PERFORMANCE CHECKLIST

Skill 12-4   Testing visual acuity

Student: _____

Date: __ _____

	Satisfactory	Unsatisfactory
1. Carries out Standard Steps A, B, C, D, and E as need indicates.	❏	❏
2. Positions person at distance of 20 feet from eye chart.	❏	❏
3. Has patient remove corrective lens; occludes one eye.	❏	❏
4. Instructs to read lines on the chart.	❏	❏
5. Records the score.	❏	❏
6. Repeats exam for the other eye.	❏	❏
7. Repeats the test with corrective lenses, if used.	❏	❏

Pass _____

Fail _____

Comments: _____

_____

Instructor: _____

© 1994 W.B. Saunders Company. *Rambo's Nursing Skills for Clinical Practice,* fourth edition
All rights reserved.

PERFORMANCE CHECKLIST

Skill 12-5   Spoken or whispered voice test

Student: _____

Date: _____

	Satisfactory	**Unsatisfactory**
1. Carries out Standard Steps A, B, C, D, and E as appropriate.	❏	❏
2. Instructs person to cover and close both eyes.	❏	❏
3. Mask one ear.	❏	❏
4. Asks person to raise hand when he hears a word and then to repeat the word.	❏	❏
5. Stands at a distance and speaks or whispers several words toward ear being tested.	❏	❏
6. Repeat the test for the other ear.	❏	❏
7. Carries out Standard Steps X, Y, and Z.	❏	❏

Pass _____

Fail _____

Comments: _____

_____

Instructor: _____

© 1994 W.B. Saunders Company. *Rambo's Nursing Skills for Clinical Practice,* fourth edition
All rights reserved.

PERFORMANCE CHECKLIST

Skill 12-6   Watch tick test

Student: _____

Date: _____

	Satisfactory	Unsatisfactory
1. Carries out Standard Steps A, B, C, D, and E as appropriate.	❏	❏
2. Seats person in a quiet area.	❏	❏
3. Masks ear not being tested.	❏	❏
4. Holds ticking watch next to ear being tested.	❏	❏
5. Asks person to indicate when he can no longer hear the watch.	❏	❏
6. Moves watch away until ticking is no longer heard.	❏	❏
7. Records the greatest distance at which watch can be heard.	❏	❏
8. Tests other ear.	❏	❏
9. Carries out Standard Steps X, Y, and Z.	❏	❏

Pass _____

Fail _____

Comments: _____

_____

Instructor: _____

© 1994 W.B. Saunders Company. *Rambo's Nursing Skills for Clinical Practice,* fourth edition
All rights reserved.

PERFORMANCE CHECKLIST

Skill 12-7   Weber's test

Student: _____

Date: _____

	Satisfactory	**Unsatisfactory**
1. Carries out Standard Steps A, B, C, D, and E as appropriate.	❏	❏
2. Seats person in a quiet area.	❏	❏
3. Strikes the tuning fork so it commences vibrating.	❏	❏
4. Places tuning fork on person's midforehead.	❏	❏
5. Asks person to describe the sound and whether it is louder in one ear than the other.	❏	❏
6. Records the result.	❏	❏

Pass _____

Fail _____

Comments: _____

_____

Instructor: _____

© 1994 W.B. Saunders Company. *Rambo's Nursing Skills for Clinical Practice,* fourth edition
All rights reserved.

PERFORMANCE CHECKLIST

Skill 12-8   Rinne test

Student: _____

Date: _____

	Satisfactory	**Unsatisfactory**
1. Carries out Standard Steps A, B, C, D, and E as appropriate.	❏	❏
2. Seats person in a quiet area.	❏	❏
3. Masks one ear.	❏	❏
4. Strikes tuning fork to commence vibrating.	❏	❏
5. Places the base of the tuning fork on the mastoid process behind ear being tested.	❏	❏
6. Asks person to indicate when sound is no longer heard.	❏	❏
7. Places prongs of the tuning fork in front of the ear canal when person indicates he no longer can hear sound.	❏	❏
8. Notes length of time sound is heard.	❏	❏
9. Repeats the test for the other ear.	❏	❏
10. Records results.	❏	❏

Pass _____

Fail _____

Comments: _____

_____

Instructor: _____

© 1994 W.B. Saunders Company. *Rambo's Nursing Skills for Clinical Practice,* fourth edition
All rights reserved.

Suggested Clinical Activities

1. Practice performing an initial physical and psychosocial assessment on classmates and family members. Organize your approach so that it will be in a consistent order each time you perform such an assessment.

2. Practice the neurological "check" on at least four people.

3. Review in your mind the equipment and steps needed to prepare a patient for a physical examination and to assist a physician with the examination.

4. On the hospital unit to which you are assigned, review the procedure for setting up and assisting the physician with a proctosigmoidoscopy examination, and for a pelvic examination and pap smear.

5. Practice the various hearing tests on three peers in the nursing skill laboratory.

6. Make up index cards to guide you when doing a complete physical and psychosocial assessment. Use an outline format. Utilize these cards when you are in the clinical setting.

© 1994 W.B. Saunders Company. *Rambo's Nursing Skills for Clinical Practice,* fourth edition
All rights reserved.

Chapter 13

Diagnostic Tests and Procedures and Patient Preparation

LEARNING ACTIVITIES

I. Match the term in Column I with the definition in Column II.

Column I

_____ 1. angiography
_____ 2. bronchoscopy
_____ 3. culture
_____ 4. CT scan
_____ 5. cystoscopy
_____ 6. endoscopy
_____ 7. IVP
_____ 8. lumbar puncture
_____ 9. Pap smear
_____10. proctosigmoidoscopy
_____11. thoracentesis
_____12. venipuncture

Column II

a. examination of the rectum and sigmoid colon with a proctoscope.

b. computerized tomography scan.

c. inspection of the interior of the tracheobronchial tree through a bronchoscope.

d. insertion of a needle into the sub-arachnoid space between the lumbar vertebrae to withdraw cerebrospinal fluid.

e. examination of a body cavity via a tube.

f. radiography of an artery after injection with a contrast medium into the bloodstream.

g. growing organisms in a laboratory culture medium.

h. examination of the bladder through a a cystoscope.

i. intravenous pyelogram.

j. laboratory test to determine cervical (or other) cancer.

k. insertion of a needle into a vein to withdraw blood.

l. insertion of a needle into the pleural space to withdraw fluid or air or to instill medication.

© 1994 W.B. Saunders Company. *Rambo's Nursing Skills for Clinical Practice,* fourth edition
All rights reserved.

II. Fill in the blank(s) with the appropriate word or phrase.

1. Diagnostic tests are performed to aid in the _____ of disease.

2. Magnetic resonance imaging is a _____ method of visualizing

   _____ without the use of contrast media or ionizing radiation.

3. Sonography uses _____ to outline structures.

4. Cultures and smears are taken to help determine _____.

5. _____ tests are performed to study the _____.

6. Certain _____ may cause a sharp fall in leukocytes.

7. The test performed to monitor heparin therapy is _____.

8. The _____ is used to adjust dosages of oral anticoagulant
   drugs such as sodium wafarin (Coumadin).

9. The normal range of hemoglobin for the male is _____ and for the female it is _____.

10. A normal platelet count is between _____.

11. A normal urine specimen does NOT contain _____

    _____.

12. Blood chemistry tests reveal changes in _____ reactions in the body.

13. Two blood chemistry tests that give an indication of kidney function are _____

    and _____.

14. KUB stands for _____.

15. Common xrays of the GI system include an _____ and
    a _____.

© 1994 W.B. Saunders Company. *Rambo's Nursing Skills for Clinical Practice*, fourth edition
All rights reserved.

16. Mammograms are special xrays of the _____ and are done with

_____.

17. Chest xrays are usually done with the patient in an _____ position.

18. The test normally done when gallbladder problems are suspected is _____.

19. A barium swallow and upper GI series takes about _____ minutes.

20. After a barium xray it is important that the patient be given a _____.

21. After any diagnostic test that utilizes a contrast medium or dye of some sort, the patient is encouraged to

_____.

22. One non-invasive test of heart function is the _____.

23. A non-invasive cardiac test utilizing exercise is the _____ test.

24. Cardiac catheterization is done to determine the function of the _____

_____.

25. An ERCP, _____,

is done to identify _____.

26. A Class IV Pap smear is _____.

27. A wound culture is performed to determine the _____ and then a _____

test is done to identify _____.

28. Before a bone marrow aspiration is done, the patient should be given a _____.

29. A paracentesis is performed to _____ or to initiate

_____.

30. An EEG is done to localize and diagnose _____ _____.

© 1994 W.B. Saunders Company. *Rambo's Nursing Skills for Clinical Practice,* fourth edition
All rights reserved.

III. Take the post-test included at the end of the chapter in the text.

© 1994 W.B. Saunders Company. *Rambo's Nursing Skills for Clinical Practice,* fourth edition
All rights reserved.

PERFORMANCE CHECKLIST

Skill 13-1   Mouth and Throat Culture

Student: _____

Date: _____

	Satisfactory	Unsatisfactory
1. Carries out Standard Steps A, B, C, D, and E as appropriate.	❏	❏
2. Maintains sterile technique while swabbing nose and/or throat.	❏	❏
3. Activates culture medium in tube.	❏	❏
4. Labels culture tube.	❏	❏
5. Fills out laboratory requisition slip.	❏	❏
6. Transports specimen to laboratory.	❏	❏
7. Documents procedure and carries out Standard Steps X, Y, and Z.	❏	❏

Pass _____

Fail _____

Comments: _____

_____

Instructor: _____

© 1994 W.B. Saunders Company. *Rambo's Nursing Skills for Clinical Practice,* fourth edition
All rights reserved.

PERFORMANCE CHECKLIST

Skill 13-2   Wound culture

Student: _____

Date: _____

	Satisfactory	Unsatisfactory
1. Carries out Standard Steps A, B, C, D, and E as appropriate.	❏	❏
2. Removes soiled dressing aseptically.	❏	❏
3. Cleanses area around the wound.	❏	❏
4. Swabs the wound with a sterile applicator.	❏	❏
5. Places applicator in culture tube.	❏	❏
6. Applies sterile dressing.	❏	❏
7. Activates culture medium in tube.	❏	❏
8. Labels the culture tube.	❏	❏
9. Fills out laboratory requisition.	❏	❏
10. Delivers specimen to laboratory.	❏	❏
11. Documents procedure and carries out Standard Steps X, Y, and Z.	❏	❏

Pass _____

Fail _____

Comments: _____

_____

Instructor: _____

© 1994 W.B. Saunders Company. *Rambo's Nursing Skills for Clinical Practice,* fourth edition
All rights reserved.

PERFORMANCE CHECKLIST

Skill 13-3   Urine culture

Student: _____

Date: _____

	Satisfactory	Unsatisfactory
1. Carries out Standard Steps A, B, C, D and E as appropriate.	❏	❏
2. Clears catheter tubing of urine and clamps catheter for 15–20 minutes.	❏	❏
3. Washes hands and dons gloves.	❏	❏
4. Cleanses the injection port and withdraws 2–5 mL of urine using sterile syringe and small gauge needle.	❏	❏
5. Wipes port with alcohol swab after withdrawing needle.	❏	❏
6. Places urine in sterile specimen cup using sterile technique.	❏	❏
7. Disposes of needle and syringe in sharps container.	❏	❏
8. Removes gloves and washes hands.	❏	❏
9. Labels the specimen.	❏	❏
10. Fills out requisition slip.	❏	❏
11. Delivers specimen to laboratory or refrigerates specimen.	❏	❏
12. Documents procedure and carries out Standard Steps X, Y, and Z.	❏	❏

Pass: _____

Fail: _____

Comments: _____

_____

Instructor: _____

© 1994 W.B. Saunders Company. *Rambo's Nursing Skills for Clinical Practice,* fourth edition
All rights reserved.

PERFORMANCE CHECKLIST

Skill 13-4   Assisting with a Pap smear

Student: _____

Date: _____

	Satisfactory	**Unsatisfactory**
1. Carries out Standard Steps A, B, C, D, and E as need indicates; prepares the equipment and supplies.	❏	❏
2. Identifies slides appropriately.	❏	❏
3. Positions and drapes patient.	❏	❏
4. Dons gloves and fixes tissue on slides.	❏	❏
5. Repositions patient after procedure; offers tissues or cleanses perineum.	❏	❏
6. Places slides in transport container.	❏	❏
7. Removes gloves and washes hands.	❏	❏
8. Fills out laboratory requisition.	❏	❏
9. Routes specimens to laboratory.	❏	❏
10. Documents procedure and carries out Standard Steps X, Y, and Z.	❏	❏

Pass _____

Fail _____

Comments: _____

_____

Instructor: _____

© 1994 W.B. Saunders Company. *Rambo's Nursing Skills for Clinical Practice,* fourth edition
All rights reserved.

PERFORMANCE CHECKLIST

Skill 13-5   Measuring blood glucose with a glucometer

Student: _____

Date: _____

	Satisfactory	Unsatisfactory
1. Carries out Standard Steps A, B, C, D, and E as appropriate.	❏	❏
2. Sets up and calibrates glucometer.	❏	❏
3. Washes hands and dons gloves	❏	❏
4. Washes and dries the area to be used for finger or heel stick.	❏	❏
5. Obtains good blood supply in area before performing stick.	❏	❏
6. Utilizes automatic lancet device correctly.	❏	❏
7. Obtains free-flowing, adequately large, drop of blood.	❏	❏
8. Places drop of blood on appropriate area for test: reagent strip; reading platform.	❏	❏
9. Wipes puncture site and stanches bleeding.	❏	❏
10. Times test accurately.	❏	❏
11. Takes readings and records in appropriate location.	❏	❏
12. Carries out Standard Steps X, Y, Z; turns off machine and cleans up equipment.	❏	❏
13. Removes gloves and washes hands.	❏	❏

Pass _____

Fail _____

Comments: _____

_____

Instructor: _____

© 1994 W.B. Saunders Company. *Rambo's Nursing Skills for Clinical Practice,* fourth edition
All rights reserved.

PERFORMANCE CHECKLIST

Skill 13-6   Assisting with a proctosigmoidoscopy

Student: _____

Date: _____

	Satisfactory	Unsatisfactory
1. Institutes dietary regimen 24 hours before test.	❏	❏
2. Carries out Standard Steps A, B, C, D, and E as need indicates.	❏	❏
3. Administers pre-test care: laxatives, enemas.	❏	❏
4. Has patient void before procedure.	❏	❏
5. Sets up equipment and checks light on proctosigmoidoscope and checks suction.	❏	❏
6. Positions patient appropriately on table.	❏	❏
7. Offers encouragement and support to patient during exam.	❏	❏
8. Repositions patient after exam.	❏	❏
9. Prepares tissue specimens appropriately and sends to laboratory.	❏	❏
10. Makes patient comfortable in own room.	❏	❏
11. Documents procedure and carries out Standard Steps X,Y,and Z.	❏	❏

Pass _____

Fail _____

Comments: _____

_____

Instructor: _____

© 1994 W.B. Saunders Company. *Rambo's Nursing Skills for Clinical Practice,* fourth edition
All rights reserved.

Suggested Clinical Activities

1. Scan an assigned patient's diagnostic test results; determine if the test result was normal or abnormal. Look at each part of the CBC to see if it is within normal range.

2. Determine which tests would most likely be ordered for the following patients:
   a. a man with jaundice.
   b. a woman with nausea and abdominal pain.
   c. a man with signs of kidney failure.
   d. a woman with a fever and malaise.

3. Prepare to teach a patient about the following tests:
   a. abdominal sonogram
   b. MRI of the knee
   c. upper G. I. and Barium enema
   d. colonoscopy
   e. glucose tolerance test

4. Plan after test care for the following patients:
   a. Mr. Soda who had a colonoscopy
   b. Mrs. White who had an Upper G. I. and Barium Enema
   c. Mr. Horton who had a myelogram and a lumbar puncture.

II. Take the post-test included at the end of the chapter in the text.

© 1994 W.B. Saunders Company. *Rambo's Nursing Skills for Clinical Practice,* fourth edition
All rights reserved.

Chapter 14

Documentation of Nursing Care

LEARNING ACTIVITIES

EXERCISE 1

DIRECTIONS: Select the phrase from Column 2 that best describes the words in Column 1. Write the letter designating that phrase in the blank space in Column 1.

Column 1	Column 2
____ 1. coughs up material	a. hyperpnea
____ 2. unpleasant	b. radiating
____ 3. pungent	c. halitosis
____ 4. sudden attacks of coughing	d. stertorous
____ 5. partly conscious	respirations
____ 6. spreads to areas	e. productive
____ 7. unpleasant breath	f. orthopnea
____ 8. localized muscle	g. lethargic
____ contraction	h. aromatic
____ 9. taking in air	i. inspiration
____10. cannot breathe lying down	j. foul
	k. spasm
	l. paroxysmal

EXERCISE 2

DIRECTIONS: Read the following situation and chart using the source-oriented or narrative charting format. Remember to include information characterizing the patient's symptoms.

SITUATION: Charlie Reid is a 50-year-old hospital pharmacist who was admitted 3 hours earlier with complaints of substernal chest pain and shortness of breath associated with the pain. At 9:00 AM Mr. Reid stated that he was having severe, squeezing chest pain that traveled to his left arm and jaw. He was sweating and stated that he could hardly breathe. His BP was 168/88, P 124, and R 26. The physician was called at 0900 and he ordered Nitroglycerine 0.4 mg to be given sublingually. At 0905 Nitroglycerine 0.4 mg was given as ordered and Mr. Reid stated that he no longer had chest pain. Vital signs: BP 140/60, P 118, R 22. Also, his skin was no longer diaphoretic.

_____
_____
_____
_____
_____
_____
_____
_____

Note: Did you chart all essential details? Review your terminology and abbreviations. Are they accurate and precise? Can the reader identify your intervention for the patient and the evaluation of care?

II. Take the post-test included at the end of the chapter in the text.

© 1994 W.B. Saunders Company. *Rambo's Nursing Skills for Clinical Practice,* fourth edition
All rights reserved.

PERFORMANCE CHECKLIST

Skill: 14-1 Documentation

Student: _____

Date: _____

	Satisfactory	Unsatisfactory
1. Uses correct documentation style.	❏	❏
2. Uses correct forms.	❏	❏
3. Charts information in correct location.	❏	❏
4. Uses black/blue ink.	❏	❏
5. Writes legibly.	❏	❏
6. Corrects errors appropriately.	❏	❏
7. Dates and times entry.	❏	❏
8. Does not duplicate information.	❏	❏
9. Keeps information brief and concise, but complete.	❏	❏
10. Uses correct abbreviations.	❏	❏
11. Uses correct signature.	❏	❏
12. Terms used are objective and descriptive.	❏	❏
13. Documents after service is rendered.	❏	❏
14. Does not leave blank lines in charting.	❏	❏
15. Documents travel to other departments by patient.	❏	❏
16. Documents assessment data.	❏	❏
17. Identifies problems.	❏	❏
18. Documents nursing actions performed.	❏	❏
19. Evaluates effectiveness of actions.	❏	❏
20. Notes routine care on flow sheets where appropriate.	❏	❏

Pass _____

Fail _____

Comments: _____

_____

Instructor: _____

© 1994 W.B. Saunders Company. *Rambo's Nursing Skills for Clinical Practice,* fourth edition
All rights reserved.

Suggested Clinical Activities

1. Read the nurses notes that other staff nurses have written, with the charge/primary nurse's permission, and identify four characteristics of good documentation.

2. Review each of the flow sheet chart forms for the types of information that is to be recorded.

3. Write out nurse's notes daily on each assigned patient, trying to obtain a "picture" of the patient for someone else reading the note. Edit your notes to make them more concise and objective.

4. Review the hospital charting/documentation manual for specific requirements of the assigned facility that may vary from what you learned in lecture or from texts.

© 1994 W.B. Saunders Company. *Rambo's Nursing Skills for Clinical Practice,* fourth edition
All rights reserved.

Chapter 15

Admission, Transfer, and Discharge

LEARNING ACTIVITIES

I. Fill in the blank(s) with the appropriate word(s) or phrase.

1. List three types of admissions within the hospital setting:

    a. _____

    b. _____

    c. _____

2. Four types of information included in the orientation of the patient to the nursing unit include:

    a. _____

    b. _____

    c. _____

    d. _____

3. Briefly describe the nursing procedure for transferring a patient to another unit within the hospital.

    _____

    _____

    _____

    _____

4. When admitting an elderly patient to the nursing unit, the nurse should remember that elderly patients

    _____ and may need _____

    before the admission can be completed.

5. When admitting an elderly patient is important that the nurse proceed _____ and not _____ the patient.

© 1994 W.B. Saunders Company. *Rambo's Nursing Skills for Clinical Practice,* fourth edition   205
All rights reserved.

6. When the patient has a decreased level of consciousness, the nurse must obtain the admission information from

_____ or a _____.

7. Seven types of information that can be obtained on the admission of "face" sheet in the patient's chart include:

a. _____

b. _____

c. _____

d. _____

e. _____

f. _____

g. _____

8. Upon admission to a hospital, every patient has an _____ band attached to the arm.

9. Each patient must sign a consent for _____ and _____.

10. A major reason patients are not usually allowed to keep medications brought from home with them is that

_____.

11. The information gathered during the nursing assessment is used to complete a patient _____

_____.

12. Discharge planning must begin upon _____.

13. Upon discharge, it is important that the nurse check the patient for _____

_____.

14. Every patient is given discharge _____ before departing from the unit for home or another facility.

15. Whenever a patient insists on leaving the hospital, even though his physician is not ready to discharge him, the nurse

must _____.

II. Take the post-test included at the end of the chapter in the text.

© 1994 W.B. Saunders Company. *Rambo's Nursing Skills for Clinical Practice,* fourth edition
All rights reserved.

PERFORMANCE CHECKLIST

Skill: 15-1   Admission of patient to unit

Student: _____

Date: _____

	Satisfactory	Unsatisfactory
1. Carries out Standard Steps A and B.	❏	❏
2. Prepares the room and bed; obtains and opens admit kit and arranges items.	❏	❏
3. Checks the armband for accuracy.	❏	❏
4. Obtains urine specimen if required.	❏	❏
5. Assists patient to store belongings.	❏	❏
6. Places valuables in hospital safe.	❏	❏
7. Performs the admission assessment correctly.	❏	❏
8. Explains the use of the hospital bed, TV/radio, side rails, call light system, telephone, and drapes.	❏	❏
9. Explains hospital routine and visiting hours.	❏	❏
10. Provides for patient's safety.	❏	❏
11. Answers questions.	❏	❏
12. Records data gathered.	❏	❏
13. Reports unusual findings to charge nurse and/ or physician.	❏	❏

Pass _____

Fail _____

Comments: _____

_____

Instructor: _____

© 1994 W.B. Saunders Company. *Rambo's Nursing Skills for Clinical Practice,* fourth edition
All rights reserved.

PERFORMANCE CHECKLIST

Skill 15-2   Discharge of patient from hospital

Student: _____

Date: _____

		Satisfactory	Unsatisfactory
1.	Carries out Standard Steps A and B.	❏	❏
2.	Checks discharge order.	❏	❏
3.	Explains the discharge procedure.	❏	❏
4.	Completes the discharge form.	❏	❏
5.	Returns valuables stored in the safe.	❏	❏
6.	Gives discharge instructions and provides instructions in writing as needed.	❏	❏
7.	Obtains feedback that patient understands the instructions.	❏	❏
8.	Checks patient for attached equipment and removes it.	❏	❏
9.	Helps patient pack belongings and prepares patient for discharge.	❏	❏
10.	Helps patient complete discharge procedure with business office.	❏	❏
11.	Verifies that business office has released the patient.	❏	❏
12.	Obtains a wheelchair and a cart.	❏	❏
13.	Has patient and belongings transported to discharge location.	❏	❏
14.	Returns wheelchair and cart to storage area.	❏	❏
15.	Prepares patient's room for terminal cleaning.	❏	❏
16.	Returns unused drugs to the pharmacy.	❏	❏
17.	Notes patient discharge on unit records.	❏	❏
18.	Completes patient documentation.	❏	❏

Pass _____

Fail _____

Comments: _____

_____

Instructor: _____

© 1994 W.B. Saunders Company. *Rambo's Nursing Skills for Clinical Practice,* fourth edition
All rights reserved.

PERFORMANCE CHECKLIST

Skill 15-3   Patient transfer to another unit

Student: _____

Date: _____

		Satisfactory	Unsatisfactory
1.	Identifies the patient and explains the reason for the transfer.	❑	❑
2.	Collects patient's personal belongings.	❑	❑
3.	Moves the patient to the new nursing unit.	❑	❑
4.	Reports to the receiving nurse on the new unit.	❑	❑
5.	Notes the transfer on the patient's chart.	❑	❑
6.	Returns the equipment used for transfer to the original unit storage area.	❑	❑
7.	Prepares the patient's former unit for terminal cleaning.	❑	❑

Pass _____

Fail _____

Comments: _____

_____

Instructor: _____

© 1994 W.B. Saunders Company. *Rambo's Nursing Skills for Clinical Practice,* fourth edition
All rights reserved.

PERFORMANCE CHECKLIST

Skill 15-5   Discharge by death

Student: _____

Date: _____

	Satisfactory	Unsatisfactory
1. Checks that death has been pronounced.	❑	❑
2. Performs post-mortem care of the body.	❑	❑
3. Sees that body is transported to morgue or released to the mortuary.	❑	❑
4. Collects patient's personal belongings and valuables and releases them to the next of kin.	❑	❑
5. Returns unused drugs to the pharmacy and returns equipment to Central Supply.	❑	❑
6. Completes documentation process and discharges patient from unit records.	❑	❑
7. Prepares the chart for the medical records department.	❑	❑

Pass _____

Fail _____

Comments: _____

_____

Instructor: _____

© 1994 W.B. Saunders Company. *Rambo's Nursing Skills for Clinical Practice,* fourth edition
All rights reserved.

Suggested Clinical Activities

1. Review the nursing admission assessment forms in an assigned patient's chart noting the types of information required.

2. Accompany a staff nurse who is admitting a new patient.

3. Accompany a staff nurse who is transferring a patient to another unit within the hospital.

4. Assist with receiving a transfer patient from another unit.

5. Practice the admission procedure with a peer.

6. Role play a situation in which a patient seeks to leave AMA.

© 1994 W.B. Saunders Company. *Rambo's Nursing Skills for Clinical Practice,* fourth edition
All rights reserved.

Chapter 16

Patient Teaching, Discharge Planning, and Transition to Home Care

LEARNING ACTIVITIES

I. Fill in the blank(s) with the appropriate word(s) or phrase.

1. The three routes by which people learn are:

   a. _____

   b. _____

   c. _____

2. By what route do you think you learn best? _____

3. Considering your best route of learning, what methods of study would be best for you?

   _____

   _____

   _____

4. Before planning teaching for a patient, it is necessary to _____

   _____ .

5. When teaching patients with complex learning needs, the first area to focus on is the basic _____

   _____ the patient will need to go home safely.

6. Establishing rapport is very important to the teaching process; it begins with _____

   _____ .

All rights reserved.

7. It is important to plan the teaching sessions so that there are a minimum of _____.

8. Physical blocks to learning might include _____

_____.

9. "Situational" blocks to learning often include _____.

10. It is best to plan teaching sessions for when the patient is most _____ and _____.

11. The teaching plan should be part of the nursing _____.

12. The nursing diagnosis utilized for patients who have learning needs is "_____"
    followed by the a specific such as self-administration of insulin.

13. A teaching plan is very important because _____ in teaching is important
    for retention of the information.

14. The teaching plan should be reviewed _____ for
    areas needing change.

15. Three types of resources for patient teaching and meeting patient learning needs are:

    a. _____

    b. _____

    c. _____

16. Evaluating the effectiveness of your teaching involves getting _____ from the patient regarding
    what was taught.

17. The discharge planner coordinates and arranges _____

_____.

18. When preparing the patient for home care, the nurse should provide both written and verbal instructions on

_____,and

_____.

© 1994 W.B. Saunders Company. *Rambo's Nursing Skills for Clinical Practice,* fourth edition
All rights reserved.

19. Before the patient leaves the hospital, the nurse and/or discharge planner should evaluate whether the patient will need

the assistance of a _____ for further teaching or specific care.

20. A major reason for the increased need for thorough patient teaching for the hospital patient is the decrease in

_____.

Suggested Clinical Activities

1. Determine the most frequent types of teaching needed on the unit to which you are assigned. Prepare outlines for teaching various patients on this unit.

2. Evaluate the learning needs of each assigned patient.

3. Prepare a needed teaching plan for an assigned patient.

4. Practice teaching with a peer; obtain feedback from your peer.

5. Evaluate your teaching; revise the plan as needed.

© 1994 W.B. Saunders Company. *Rambo's Nursing Skills for Clinical Practice,* fourth edition
All rights reserved.

Chapter 17

Assisting with Spiritual Care

LEARNING ACTIVITIES

I. Fill in the blank(s) with the appropriate word(s) or phrase.

1. As a nurse it is important to respect a person's spiritual beliefs because these beliefs help _____ the person in times of illness and stress.

2. The nurse can help patients spiritually by _____ to them and helping them

   _____ their feelings.

3. The nurse needs to remember that patients have a _____ to their feelings, whatever they may be.

4. A part of spiritual care by the nurse is asking the patient if a _____, _____,

   _____ or _____ is desired.

5. The two things that are essential for the nurse to adequately assist patients with issues of spirituality are:

   a. _____

   b. _____

6. The three main religions common in the United States are:

   a. _____

   b. _____

   c. _____

7. All three of these religions stress moral codes that reject:

   a. _____

   b. _____

   c. _____

   d. _____

All rights reserved.

8. Jewish dietary laws forbid the mixing of _____ and _____ in the same utensil.

9. Orthodox Jews do not eat _____ or _____.

10. Jewish parents have their male children _____.

11. Within the Christian religion, the Catholics believe that sins are forgiven by _____

_____

12. The Catholic religion prohibits the practice of _____, except for _____.

13. A pertinent belief of Jehovah's Witnesses affecting health care of an individual is that _____

_____ is not permitted.

14. Christian Scientists believe that sickness, evil and sin are not of God but of the _____.

15. For Christian Scientists, healing of the body and mind is accomplished through _____ and

_____.

16. Two things prohibited in the Islamic religion are _____ and _____.

17. Islamic believers are required to _____ a day.

18. The main religious day of the week for Islam is _____.

19. A practice that Judaism and Islam have in common is that _____

_____.

20. Nurses sometimes will need to assist with sacraments such as _____,

_____, or _____.

II. Take the post-test included at the end of the chapter in the text.

© 1994 W.B. Saunders Company. *Rambo's Nursing Skills for Clinical Practice,* fourth edition
All rights reserved.

PERFORMANCE CHECKLIST

Skill 17-1 Assisting with Holy Communion or other sacraments

Student: _____

Date: _____

	Satisfactory	Unsatisfactory
1. Provides for toileting and washing of hands and face.	❑	❑
2. Prepares work area.	❑	❑
3. Provides for privacy for patient and clergyman.	❑	❑
4. After sacrament is complete, tidies area, makes patient comfortable, and documents procedure.	❑	❑

Pass _____

Fail _____

Comments: _____

_____

Instructor: _____

© 1994 W.B. Saunders Company. *Rambo's Nursing Skills for Clinical Practice,* fourth edition
All rights reserved.

PERFORMANCE CHECKLIST

Skill 17-2   Performing or assisting with Holy Baptism

Student: _____

Date: _____

	Satisfactory	Unsatisfactory
1. Calls clergyman if time permits.	❑	❑
2. Provides work space for baptism tray; sets up basin with holy water.	❑	❑
3. Stands by during baptism or baptizes patient.	❑	❑
4. Tidies area and makes patient comfortable.	❑	❑
5. Cleans and returns equipment to storage.	❑	❑
6. Documents procedure.	❑	❑

Pass   _____

Fail   _____

Comments: _____

_____

Instructor: _____

© 1994 W.B. Saunders Company. *Rambo's Nursing Skills for Clinical Practice,* fourth edition
All rights reserved.

Suggested Clinical Activities

1. Interview the hospital Chaplain, inquiring about the specifics of how to contact a Chaplain, ideas for suggesting a Chaplain visit, ways in which a Chaplain can help a patient, etc.

2. Perform a spiritual assessment on an assigned patient.

3. Examine your own spiritual values and determine what you do and do not believe within the common beliefs of the three most common religions in the United States.

© 1994 W.B. Saunders Company. *Rambo's Nursing Skills for Clinical Practice,* fourth edition
All rights reserved.

Chapter 18

Care of the Terminally Ill Patient and the Family

LEARNING ACTIVITIES

I. Complete the following sentences with the correct word from the vocabulary list.

Vocabulary

autopsy	pathologist
coroner	pathology
deceased	postmortem
morgue	rigor mortis
next of kin	shroud

1. When a patient has expired, the nurse performs _____ care.

2. Permission for an autopsy, unless required by law, must be obtained from the _____.

3. The person who rules as to the cause of death in questionable cases is the _____.

4. After death, the nurse prepares the body for the morgue and wraps it in a _____.

5. Several hours after death a process called _____ begins which causes the body to stiffen.

6. Unless mortuary arrangements have been made, the body of a patient who has died in the hospital is stored in the

   _____.

7. Examinations of tissues removed from a body after death to determine the cause of death are performed by a

   _____.

8. When a patient has died, he is said to be _____.

9. Examination of a dead body to determine the cause of death is called an _____.

10. The study of the cause of disease is _____.

All rights reserved.

II. Fill in the blank(s) with the appropriate word(s) or phrases.

1. All nurses must come to terms with the _____ of death.

2. Approximately _____ per cent of deaths in this country occur in hospitals.

3. An alternative to care of the terminally ill in the hospital is _____ care.

4. The purpose of hospice care is:

    _____

    _____

    _____

5. The fundamental belief in hospice care is that death is _____.

6. Three areas that are the focus of hospice care are:

    a. _____

    b. _____

    c. _____

7. The five stages of the grief process for the dying patient and the family are:

    a. _____

    b. _____

    c. _____

    d. _____

    e. _____

8. Give an example of a statement of action that would indicate that the dying person was in each of these phases of grief.

    a. Denial: _____

    b. Anger: _____

    c. Bargaining: _____

    d. Depression: _____

    e. Acceptance: _____

© 1994 W.B. Saunders Company. *Rambo's Nursing Skills for Clinical Practice,* fourth edition
All rights reserved.

9. Although the nurse knows that family members also go through these stages of grief, it is important to remember that no two family members _____.

10. The three main fears commonly expressed by the dying patient are:

    a. _____

    b. _____

    c. _____

11. Most patients who are very near death do not want_____.

12. One thing that the family can do that is helpful to the patient who is dying is to talk about the _____.

13. _____ beliefs can provide considerable support for the patient who is dying.

14. Nurses quickly learn that issues connected with the care of the terminally ill are not all cut and dried and that there are many _____.

15. One factor that has increased the bioethical questions is the increase in _____ that makes the extension of life by artificial means possible.

16. Most states now allow patients to write _____ expressing wishes regarding the withholding of life-sustaining measures in the event of terminal illness or injury.

17. It is important that the dying patient have time with loved ones for _____.

18. The state requires a _____ for every person who dies.

19. Nurses and physicians are now responsible for speaking to the patient and/or family about _____ when the patient is considered terminal.

20. A death occurring in the hospital within _____ is investigated by the coroner.

III. Take the post-test included at the end of the chapter in the text.

© 1994 W.B. Saunders Company. *Rambo's Nursing Skills for Clinical Practice,* fourth edition
All rights reserved.

PERFORMANCE CHECKLIST

Skill 18-1   Giving postmortem care

Student: _____

Date: _____

	Satisfactory	Unsatisfactory
1. Prepares equipment, washes hands, follows universal precautions, provides privacy.	❏	❏
2. Positions body supine, in proper alignment, with head slightly elevated.	❏	❏
3. Removes or secures all tubes and lines.	❏	❏
4. Cleans body appropriately.	❏	❏
5. Changes soiled dressings.	❏	❏
6. Places clean gown on body and straightens room.	❏	❏
7. Allows viewing time for family; remains in room to offer emotional support.	❏	❏
8. Follows agency procedure for preparing the body in the shroud for the morgue.	❏	❏
9. Transports the body to the morgue.	❏	❏
10. Documents the procedure correctly.	❏	❏

Pass _____

Fail _____

Comments: _____

_____

Instructor: _____

© 1994 W.B. Saunders Company. *Rambo's Nursing Skills for Clinical Practice,* fourth edition
All rights reserved.

Suggested Clinical Activities

1. Imagine you have just been diagnosed with a terminal illness. Think about what you would want to do with your remaining days. How would you go about getting your "affairs in order?"

2. Devise a will and plan your own funeral.

3. Accompany a nurse who is going to give postmortem care.

4. Role play with a peer measures to support a grieving family member.

© 1994 W.B. Saunders Company. *Rambo's Nursing Skills for Clinical Practice,* fourth edition
All rights reserved.

Chapter 19

Comfort Measures

LEARNING ACTIVITIES

I. Insert the vocabulary word that best fits the blank in the sentence. Vocabulary agonist distraction imagery noxious analgesic

1. Nancy's mother has brought a hand-held video game to help control pain. This would be pain control by

   _____.

2. Tom had surgery yesterday and is in pain; he requests an _____.

3. The nurse asks Mary to focus on the snorkeling adventure she had last summer while she is undergoing a bone biopsy.

   This pain control technique is called _____.

4. Intramuscular injections often cause a _____ pain.

5. An _____ is a drug which binds to a cellular receptor intended for another substance, preventing the action of that substance while producing a favorable physiologic response.

II. Fill in the blank(s) with the correct word(s) or phrase.

1. The reason that objective assessment of pain is very difficult is because _____.

2. Physiologically speaking pain is _____.

3. According to the gate control theory of pain, massage helps relieve pain by _____

4. Per the gate control theory, keeping the mind very active helps control pain by _____
   _____.

5. Relaxation techniques can sometimes help decrease pain by decreasing anxiety which in turn _____
   _____.

6. Like morphine, _____ attach to nerve ending narcotic receptors and _____ pain transmission.

7. According to pain specialists, pain is _____.

8. Pain perception and pain tolerance _____ from person to person.

9. Three things that often increase pain perception in people are

   a. _____

   b. _____

   c. _____

10. The three basic categories of medications for pain relief are:
   a. _____

   b. _____

   c. _____

11. Oral medications are generally used for _____ pain.

12. A new form of time-release morphine is being used orally to control _____ and _____ pain.

13. Patients using PCA generally use less pain medication; this is probably because_____ _____.

14. PCA can be used via _____ or _____.

15. Patients receiving epidural anesthesia often are placed on _____.

16. When a patient requests pain medication, the nurse must: check _____ _____.

17. _____ after giving pain medication is very important to determine the effectiveness of the medication.

18. When utilizing heat for control of pain, heat-producing equipment such as a K-pad must have a physician's order, but _____ can usually be applied at the nurse's discretion.

19. Heat treatments are usually for a duration of _____.

© 1994 W.B. Saunders Company. *Rambo's Nursing Skills for Clinical Practice,* fourth edition
All rights reserved.

20. Three uses of cold for pain or discomfort are:

   a. _____

   b. _____

   c. _____

21. A device that can help relieve abdominal or breast pain is a _____.

22. One of the oldest forms of pain relief is _____.

23. TENS, _____, acts to _____

   the pain sensation.

24. A pain control measure used by many patients at home, especially for muscle pain, is a _____

   _____.

25. Distraction is used to alleviate pain by _____.

26. Progressive _____ techniques help many patients with chronic pain go to sleep at night.

27. With the use of biofeedback machines, the patient can be taught _____ which help decrease pain.

28. _____ is another method used to teach relaxation techniques and control pain in some individuals.

29. Guided imagery essentially helps control pain by using the mind to _____.

30. _____ helps the patient control pain by focusing on one point, sound, or pattern, thereby diverting attention away from the pain.

III. Take the post-test included at the end of the chapter in the text.

© 1994 W.B. Saunders Company. *Rambo's Nursing Skills for Clinical Practice,* fourth edition
All rights reserved.

PERFORMANCE CHECKLIST

Skill 19-1   Initial assessment of patient pain

Student: _____

Date: _____

	Satisfactory	Unsatisfactory
1. Carries out Standard Steps A, B, C, D, and E as need indicates.	❑	❑
2. Provides for pain relief prior to full assessment if appropriate.	❑	❑
3. Performs assessment.	❑	❑
a. Has the patient describe the type(s) of pain being experienced.	❑	❑
b. Numbers the location(s) on the human figure sketch on the assessment form.	❑	❑
c. Writes the description(s) as given by the patient in the assessment notes, numbered as on the sketch.	❑	❑
d. Asks the patient to describe any other regularly occurring pain that might not be present at the moment, and records as above.	❑	❑
4. Determines what pain relief measures have been effective in the past.	❑	❑
5. Actively listens to the patient's questions and concerns regarding pain and its treatment, and communicates these with other health team members as appropriate.	❑	❑
6. Plans a team conference for the patient with complex needs.	❑	❑
7. Carries out Standard Steps X, Y, and Z.	❑	❑

Pass _____

Fail _____

Comments: _____

_____

Instructor: _____

© 1994 W.B. Saunders Company. *Rambo's Nursing Skills for Clinical Practice,* fourth edition
All rights reserved.

PERFORMANCE CHECKLIST

Skill 19-2   Ongoing assessment of patient pain; Use of pain rating scales

Student: _____

Date: _____

	Satisfactory	Unsatisfactory
1. Carries out Standard Steps A, B, C, D, and E as need indicates.	❏	❏
2. Selects one or more possible pain rating scales based on the patient's age and ability to understand.	❏	❏
3. Explains use of Pain Scales to the patient and allows the patient to participate in the selection.	❏	❏
4. Teaches the patient to use the scale.	❏	❏
5. Determines through discussion and return demonstration that the patient understands the use of the scale.	❏	❏
6. Provides patient with a copy of the scale and any necessary tools.	❏	❏
7. Notes on the care plan the pain rating scale selected.	❏	❏
8. Reevaluates patient's pain at intervals throughout the shift using the scale.		
a. Determines degree of pain and selects the appropriate intervention(s).	❏	❏
b. Evaluates the effectiveness of analgesia.	❏	❏
c. Answers questions and reinstructs patient in use of scale as needed.	❏	❏
9. Utilizes Patient Pain Flow Sheet or other appropriate form as designated by the agency.	❏	❏
10. Carries out Standard Steps X, Y, and Z.	❏	❏

Pass _____

Fail _____

Comments: _____

_____

© 1994 W.B. Saunders Company. *Rambo's Nursing Skills for Clinical Practice,* fourth edition
All rights reserved.

PERFORMANCE CHECKLIST

Skill 19-3   Administration of PRN pain medication

Student: _____

Date: _____

	Satisfactory	Unsatisfactory
1. Carries out Standard Steps A, B, C, D, and E as need indicates.	❏	❏
2. Receives patient's report of pain using selected pain rating scale.	❏	❏
3. Reviews patient medication record for available analgesic(s).	❏	❏
4. Selects and administers appropriate analgesic as determined by time lapse since last dose, patient input on current analgesic needs, and previous effectiveness of available medication(s).	❏	❏
a. Explains any delay in medication due to insufficient time lapse since last dose and offers alternative if available.	❏	❏
b. Reports to the physician if dosage or intervals inadequate to control the patient's pain.	❏	❏
5. Returns in 45 minutes to 1 hour following medication administration and assesses effectiveness using pain scale.	❏	❏
6. Utilizes appropriate non-medicinal pain relief measures in conjunction with analgesic medications.	❏	❏
7. Carries out Standard Steps X, Y, and Z.	❏	❏

Pass _____

Fail _____

Comments: _____

_____

Instructor: _____

© 1994 W.B. Saunders Company. *Rambo's Nursing Skills for Clinical Practice,* fourth edition
All rights reserved.

PERFORMANCE CHECKLIST

Skill 19-4   Administering a back rub

Student: _____

Date: _____

	Satisfactory	**Unsatisfactory**
1. Carries out Standard Steps A, B, C, D, and E as need indicates.	❑	❑
2. Elevates side rails and raises bed to an appropriate height.	❑	❑
3. Lowers rail only on side of bed where standing during back rub and raises rail whenever stepping away from bedside.	❑	❑
4. Assists patient into prone position.	❑	❑
5. Uses bed covers as drape to cover patient from waist down for privacy and warmth.	❑	❑
6. Performs back rub.		
a. Warms lotion in palms of hands before applying.	❑	❑
b. Applies lotion using long gently firm strokes, avoiding open wounds and any areas of pressure injury.	❑	❑
c. Rubs in the lotion using short, circular strokes.	❑	❑
d. Uses *tapotement* technique only on patients with good muscle tone and skeletal integrity.	❑	❑
7. Prepares patient for sleep following back rub.		
a. Assists patient to position of comfort.	❑	❑
b. Raises side rail and lowers the bed.	❑	❑
8. Carries out Standard Steps X, Y, and Z.	❑	❑

Pass _____

Fail _____

Comments: _____

_____

Instructor: _____

© 1994 W.B. Saunders Company. *Rambo's Nursing Skills for Clinical Practice,* fourth edition
All rights reserved.

Suggested Clinical Activities

1. Observe a nurse setting up a PCA pump and go with her while she instructs the patient and attaches it to the IV line.

2. Practice alternative pain control techniques for a family member of friend for relief of a headache, muscle spasm, etc.

3. Practice back massage techniques on a family member or friend until you have confidence in your massage technique.

4. Develop your own guided imagery "script" for use with patients.

© 1994 W.B. Saunders Company. *Rambo's Nursing Skills for Clinical Practice,* fourth edition
All rights reserved.

Chapter 20

Hot and Cold Applications

LEARNING ACTIVITIES

I. Fill in the blank(s) with the correct word(s) or phrase.

1. Three purposes of applying heat to the body are:

    a. _____

    b. _____

    c. _____

2. When applying a heat treatment to an elderly patient, the nurse must be very careful as this patient's skin may _____ more quickly.

3. Heat _____ the blood vessels in the area of application.

4. Using heat to increase the blood supply in a body area does the following three things:

    a. _____

    b. _____

    c. _____

5. The maximum temperature for a heat treatment is _____ F. or _____ C.

6. One advantage of the disposal, one-time use, hot pack is that it reduces the chance of _____.

7. Home hot packs will retain their heat longer if _____ is placed over the pack.

8. Hot soaks are generally used for the _____.

9. A special type of hot soak therapy is a _____ treatment.

10. The length of time a hot compress stays hot depends on:

    a. _____

    b. _____

    c. _____

11. In the hospital, a continuous heat treatment is usually performed with the use of _____.

12. Hot water bottles are no longer used in health care facilities because of the risk of _____.

13. A heat lamp should be positioned _____ from the area to be treated.

14. The two main purposes of using cold on the body are:

    a. _____

    b. _____

15. Cold may be painful, but prolonged cold _____.

16. _____ is more effective than air as a conductor of cold.

17. When cold is applied to the skin, _____ occurs.

18. Hypothermia treatments are used to reduce body _____ and decrease _____.

19. Cold treatments may _____ the blood pressure.

20. Cold compresses remain effective for approximately _____.

21. When the patient is placed on a hypothermia blanket, the patient's_____ must be checked frequently.

22. In general, ice should never be applied_____ to the skin for an extended period.

23. Heat and cold treatments are both used to _____.

© 1994 W.B. Saunders Company. *Rambo's Nursing Skills for Clinical Practice,* fourth edition
All rights reserved.

24. When applying cold treatments, the most effective method is to apply the cold pack for _____ of every hour.

25. When a patient is receiving hypothermia treatment, the nurse should remember that a systemic effect is the shunting

   _____.

II. Take the post-test included at the end of the chapter in the text.

© 1994 W.B. Saunders Company. *Rambo's Nursing Skills for Clinical Practice,* fourth edition
All rights reserved.

PERFORMANCE CHECKLIST

Skill 20-1   Hot or cold pack application

Student: _____

Date: _____

	Satisfactory	Unsatisfactory
1. Carries out Standard Steps A, B, C, D, and E as need indicates.	❏	❏
2. Obtains appropriate type of hot or cold pack.	❏	❏
3. Prepares pack appropriately; covers pack if needed.	❏	❏
4. Assesses area to be treated.	❏	❏
5. Applies and secures pack to area to be treated.	❏	❏
6. Frequently checks patient and replaces pack as needed.	❏	❏
7. Evaluates area treated when finished.	❏	❏
8. Carries out Standard Steps X, Y, and Z.	❏	❏

Pass _____

Fail _____

Comments: _____

_____

Instructor: _____

© 1994 W.B. Saunders Company. *Rambo's Nursing Skills for Clinical Practice,* fourth edition
All rights reserved.

PERFORMANCE CHECKLIST

Skill 20-2 Application of hot soaks

Student: _____

Date: _____

	Satisfactory	Unsatisfactory
1. Carries out Standard Steps A, B, C, D, and E as need indicates.	❏	❏
2. Assesses for risk factors.	❏	❏
3. Positions patient and prepares equipment.	❏	❏
4. Prepares heated solution and checks temperature.	❏	❏
5. Immerses limb slowly into hot solution.	❏	❏
6. At end of treatment, supports limb while lifting it from basin.	❏	❏
7. Dries limb thoroughly.	❏	❏
8. Evaluates area treated.	❏	❏
9. Applies dressing if needed.	❏	❏
10. Carries out Standard Steps X, Y, and Z.	❏	❏

Pass _____

Fail _____

Comments: _____

_____

Instructor: _____

© 1994 W.B. Saunders Company. *Rambo's Nursing Skills for Clinical Practice,* fourth edition
All rights reserved.

PERFORMANCE CHECKLIST

Skill 20-3 Application of hot compresses

Student: _____

Date: _____

	Satisfactory	Unsatisfactory
1. Carries out Standard Steps A, B, C, D, and E as need indicates.	❑	❑
2. Prepares patient and area to be treated.	❑	❑
3. Heats solution and checks temperature.	❑	❑
4. Prepares hot compresses.	❑	❑
5. Maintains sterile technique if required.	❑	❑
6. Wrings out compresses with forceps if necessary.	❑	❑
7. Wraps plastic sheeting around area and encloses with towel.	❑	❑
8. Checks patient frequently; replaces compress as needed.	❑	❑
9. At end of treatment, removes compress and pats area dry; applies new dressing if needed.	❑	❑
10. Carries out Standard Steps X, Y, and Z.	❑	❑

Pass _____

Fail _____

Comments: _____

_____

Instructor: _____

© 1994 W.B. Saunders Company. *Rambo's Nursing Skills for Clinical Practice,* fourth edition
All rights reserved.

PERFORMANCE CHECKLIST

Skill 20-4   Application of Aquathermia pad (K-pad)

Student: _____

Date: _____

	Satisfactory	Unsatisfactory
1. Carries out Standard Steps A, B, C, D, and E as need indicates.	❏	❏
2. Prepares Aquathermia unit and pad; covers pad.	❏	❏
3. Positions pad over designated area and secures pad in place.	❏	❏
4. Checks patient and area being treated at frequent intervals.	❏	❏
5. When treatment is finished, removes pad and turns off unit.	❏	❏
6. Carries out Standard Steps X, Y, and Z.	❏	❏

Pass   _____

Fail   _____

Comments: _____

_____

Instructor: _____

© 1994 W.B. Saunders Company. *Rambo's Nursing Skills for Clinical Practice,* fourth edition
All rights reserved.

PERFORMANCE CHECKLIST

Skill 20-5   Application of an electric heating pad

Student: _____

Date: _____

	Satisfactory	Unsatisfactory
1. Carries out Standard Steps A, B, C, D, and E as need indicates.	❏	❏
2. Plugs in unit and sets on "low".	❏	❏
3. Covers pad.	❏	❏
4. Positions pad on area to be treated.	❏	❏
5. Checks patient and assesses skin at frequent intervals.	❏	❏
6. When treatment time is complete, removes pad and turns it off and unplugs it.	❏	❏
7. Carries out Standard Steps X, Y, and Z.	❏	❏

Pass   _____

Fail   _____

Comments: _____

_____

Instructor: _____

© 1994 W.B. Saunders Company. *Rambo's Nursing Skills for Clinical Practice,* fourth edition
All rights reserved.

PERFORMANCE CHECKLIST

Skill 20-6   Heat lamp treatment

Student: _____

Date: _____

	Satisfactory	Unsatisfactory
1. Carries out Standard Steps A, B, C, D, and E as need indicates.	❑	❑
2. Position patient in good body alignment.	❑	❑
3. Expose the area to be treated, keeping the rest of the patient covered.	❑	❑
4. Assess area to be treated.	❑	❑
5. Position the heat lamp with the bulb 12–24 inches from area to be treated.	❑	❑
6. Plug in the cord, check wattage of bulb, and turn on the light.	❑	❑
7. Position cord to lamp so that no one will trip over it.	❑	❑
8. Places call light within reach, raises siderails if indicated.	❑	❑
9. When ordered time has elapsed, turn off lamp, re-dress wound area or cover patient.	❑	❑
10. Move heat lamp out of the way until next use.	❑	❑
11. Carries out Standard Steps X, Y, and Z.	❑	❑

Pass _____

Fail _____

Comments: _____

_____

Instructor: _____

© 1994 W.B. Saunders Company. *Rambo's Nursing Skills for Clinical Practice,* fourth edition
All rights reserved.

PERFORMANCE CHECKLIST

Skill 20-7   Hot water bottle application

Student: _____

Date: _____

	Satisfactory	**Unsatisfactory**
1. Carries out Standard Steps A, B, C, D, and E as need indicates.	❑	❑
2. Fills bottle no more than 2/3s full, expelling excess air.	❑	❑
3. Checks the temperature of the water with a bath thermometer or checks filled bottle temperature with inside of wrist.	❑	❑
4. Covers bottle and positions it over area to be treated; secures in place.	❑	❑
5. Checks on patient and temperature of bottle at frequent intervals; refills bottle when it becomes cool.	❑	❑
6. Removes, drains and airs bottle when treatment is complete.	❑	❑
7. Carries out Standard Steps X, Y, and Z.	❑	❑

Pass _____

Fail _____

Comments: _____

_____

Instructor: _____

© 1994 W.B. Saunders Company. *Rambo's Nursing Skills for Clinical Practice,* fourth edition
All rights reserved.

PERFORMANCE CHECKLIST

Skill 20-8   Sitz bath

Student: _____

Date: _____

	Satisfactory	Unsatisfactory
1. Carries out Standard Steps A, B, C, D, and E as need indicates.	❏	❏
2. Prepares sitz bath and checks water temperature.	❏	❏
3. Positions patient in sitz bath.	❏	❏
4. Checks the patient frequently assessing for dizziness or weakness.	❏	❏
5. Safely adds warm water to sitz bath as needed.	❏	❏
6. Assists patient out of sitz bath and dries perineum, supplies dry gown.	❏	❏
7. Returns patient to bed.	❏	❏
8. Carries out Standard Steps X, Y, and Z.	❏	❏

Pass _____

Fail _____

Comments: _____

_____

Instructor: _____

© 1994 W.B. Saunders Company. *Rambo's Nursing Skills for Clinical Practice,* fourth edition
All rights reserved.

PERFORMANCE CHECKLIST

Skill 20-9   Application of cold compresses

Student: _____

Date: _____

	Satisfactory	**Unsatisfactory**
1. Carries out Standard Steps A, B, C, D, and E as need indicates.	❏	❏
2. Places ice and water or special solution in basin.	❏	❏
3. Immerses gauze sponges of washcloth in iced solution.	❏	❏
4. Places plastic sheeting or underpad under area to be treated.	❏	❏
5. Wrings out compress and applies to desired area.	❏	❏
6. Checks compress frequently and replaces as needed.	❏	❏
7. Evaluates the patient and the area being treated at frequent intervals.	❏	❏
8. At end of treatment, removes compress and pats area dry.	❏	❏
9. Carries out Standard Steps X, Y, and Z.	❏	❏

Pass _____

Fail _____

Comments: _____

_____

Instructor: _____

© 1994 W.B. Saunders Company. *Rambo's Nursing Skills for Clinical Practice,* fourth edition
All rights reserved.

PERFORMANCE CHECKLIST

Skill 20-10   Application of an ice bag or ice collar

Student: _____

Date: _____

	Satisfactory	**Unsatisfactory**
1. Carries out Standard Steps A, B, C, D, and E as need indicates.	❏	❏
2. Prepares ice bag or collar and closes securely.	❏	❏
3. Positions bag on treatment area and secures in place.	❏	❏
4. Checks the patient and position of ice bag or collar at frequent intervals; replaces bag or collar when no longer cold.	❏	❏
5. At end of treatment, removes bag.	❏	❏
6. Carries out Standard Steps X, Y, and Z.	❏	❏

Pass _____

Fail _____

Comments: _____

_____

Instructor: _____

© 1994 W.B. Saunders Company. *Rambo's Nursing Skills for Clinical Practice,* fourth edition
All rights reserved.

PERFORMANCE CHECKLIST

Skill 20-11   Application of a hypothermia unit (cooling blanket)

Student: _____

Date: _____

	Satisfactory	Unsatisfactory
1. Carries out Standard Steps A, B, C, D, and E as need indicates.	❏	❏
2. Obtains and sets up hypothermia unit.	❏	❏
3. Obtains baseline vital signs.	❏	❏
4. Places patient on or between hypothermia pad(s), utilizing pad covering.	❏	❏
5. Places temperature probe into patient's rectum.	❏	❏
6. Sets temperature control for desired temperature, lowering temperature to ordered level slowly.	❏	❏
7. Wraps hands and feet as needed.	❏	❏
8. Checks patient frequently, observing for signs of impending shivering.	❏	❏
9. Checks temperature with regular thermometer every four hours; cleans temperature probe.	❏	❏
10. Monitors patient's skin condition.	❏	❏
11. When treatment is discontinued, gradually warms patient over six hours.	❏	❏
12. When treatment is over, removes pads and turns off unit.	❏	❏
13. Carries out Standard Steps X, Y, and Z.	❏	❏

Pass _____

Fail _____

Comments: _____

_____

Instructor: _____

© 1994 W.B. Saunders Company. *Rambo's Nursing Skills for Clinical Practice,* fourth edition
All rights reserved.

Suggested Clinical Activities

1. Observe a staff nurse giving a patient a heat treatment using a K-pad.

2. Determine where supplies are kept on the unit for giving hot and cold treatments such as warm or cold compresses, and ice packs.

3. Check your local pharmacy shelves for disposable types of hot and cold treatments.

4. Interview an ICU nurse about the use of hypothermia units. Discuss the nursing care involved, precautions, and instances when the device is used.

© 1994 W.B. Saunders Company. *Rambo's Nursing Skills for Clinical Practice,* fourth edition
All rights reserved.

Chapter 21

Bandages and Binders

LEARNING ACTIVITIES

I. Fill in the blank(s) with the correct word(s) or phrase.

1. Binders may be used on a wound or surgical incision to _____.

2. Pressure bandages are often used on areas of injury to _____.

3. Bandages are used on injured joints to _____ and allow for healing.

4. Dressings may sometimes be held in place by _____.

5. Binders and bandages are also used to provide _____ and increase patient comfort.

6. Breast binders are sometimes used after childbirth to _____.

7. Elastic bandages or stockings may be used on the legs of a patient to _____

   _____.

8. For the patient with an abdominal incision, an _____ will provide support, making coughing and deep breathing easier.

9. When applying a bandage, it is important that the pressure be _____

   _____.

10. If a joint is involved in bandaging it should be _____ in its normal position or

    _____.

11. Whenever a pressure bandage is applied, it is essential that periodic _____

    _____ be performed.

© 1994 W.B. Saunders Company. *Rambo's Nursing Skills for Clinical Practice,* fourth edition   279
All rights reserved.

12. Signs of impaired circulation include _____, _____,

    _____, and _____.

13. Before applying a bandage, an extremity should be _____ for _____.

14. Before applying a bandage or binder, the skin should be _____ and

    _____.

15. When wrapping a hand or foot with a bandage, it is important to place padding _____

    _____.

16. A T binder is used to apply pads or dressings to the _____.

17. Slings are used for patients who have an injury to _____.

18. A spiral bandage may be used for the following reasons:

    a. _____

    b. _____

    c. _____

19. A circular bandage is used to secure a dressing to _____.

20. A figure eight bandage is used when a _____ is included in a dressing.

II. Match the type of bandage or binder to the situation.

_____ 1. sprained ankle   a. circular bandage
_____ 2. wound on mid-lower leg   b. spiral reverse bandage
_____ 3. large abdominal incision   c. T binder
_____ 4. swollen ankle and lower leg d. figure 8 bandage
_____ 5. perineal incision   e. abdominal binder

III. Take the post-test included at the end of the chapter in the text.

© 1994 W.B. Saunders Company. *Rambo's Nursing Skills for Clinical Practice,* fourth edition
All rights reserved.

PERFORMANCE CHECKLIST

Skill 21-1 Applying an elastic or roll gauze bandage

Student: _____

Date: _____

	Satisfactory	Unsatisfactory
1. Carries out Standard Steps A, B, C, D, and E as need indicates.	❏	❏
2. Washes and dries the area to be bandaged.	❏	❏
3. Positions the patient comfortably and elevates the extremity to be bandaged.	❏	❏
4. Stands in front of patient and anchors the bandage in the appropriate location.	❏	❏
5. Uses circular turns to secure the bandage.	❏	❏
6. Bandages the area with the appropriate bandaging technique.	❏	❏
7. Applies the bandage smoothly and evenly.	❏	❏
8. Secures the bandage.	❏	❏
9. Assesses the bandage for fit and assesses for adequate circulation distal to the bandage.	❏	❏
10. Carries out Standard Steps X, Y, and Z.	❏	❏

Pass _____

Fail _____

Comments: _____

_____

Instructor: _____

© 1994 W.B. Saunders Company. *Rambo's Nursing Skills for Clinical Practice,* fourth edition
All rights reserved.

PERFORMANCE CHECKLIST

Skill 21-2   Application of a binder

Student: _____

Date: _____

	Satisfactory	Unsatisfactory
1. Carries out Standard Steps A, B, C, D, and E as need indicates.	❑	❑
2. Positions binder on or under patient in correct location.	❑	❑
3. Smoothly applies the binder.	❑	❑
4. Secures the binder with velcro fasteners or safety pins correctly.	❑	❑
5. Checks binder for proper fit.	❑	❑
6. Assesses patient and binder every two hours.	❑	❑
7. Carries out Standard Steps X, Y, and Z.	❑	❑

Pass _____

Fail _____

Comments: _____

_____

Instructor: _____

© 1994 W.B. Saunders Company. *Rambo's Nursing Skills for Clinical Practice,* fourth edition
All rights reserved.

PERFORMANCE CHECKLIST

Skill 21-3 Application of a sling (noncommercial type)

Student: _____

Date: _____

	Satisfactory	Unsatisfactory
1. Carries out Standard Steps A, B, C, D, and E as need indicates.	❑	❑
2. Places one end of triangle over shoulder on uninjured side.	❑	❑
3. Places the point of the triangle toward the elbow on the injured side.	❑	❑
4. Brings the other end over the injured arm and shoulder with the elbow bent at a right angle and the arm across the lower chest.	❑	❑
5. Ties the ends at the shoulder in a square knot.	❑	❑
6. Folds the apex neatly over the elbow toward the front and secures it with a safety pin.	❑	❑
7. Checks circulation of fingers and hand.	❑	❑
8. Carries out Standard Steps X, Y, and Z.	❑	❑

Pass _____

Fail _____

Comments: _____

_____

Instructor: _____

© 1994 W.B. Saunders Company. *Rambo's Nursing Skills for Clinical Practice,* fourth edition
All rights reserved.

Suggested Clinical Activities

1. With a classmate practice applying the following types of bandages:

   a. circular gauze bandage
   b. circular elastic bandage
   c. spiral reverse elastic bandage
   d. figure eight elastic bandage
   e. figure eight gauze bandage

2. Now practice making and applying a sling correctly.

3. Try to obtain a clinical day in the ER or the orthopedic unit and observe the way in which the nurses apply bandages to patients for various reasons.

4. In the skill lab, if available, practice applying a T-binder, abdominal binder, breast binder, and a commercial sling.

© 1994 W.B. Saunders Company. *Rambo's Nursing Skills for Clinical Practice,* fourth edition
All rights reserved.

Chapter 22

Immobility Care: Traction, Casts, Braces, and Prostheses; Special Beds and Turning Frames, Aids to Ambulation

---

LEARNING ACTIVITIES

I. *Vocabulary: Fill in the blank in the sentence with the correct vocabulary word.*

Vocabulary

bivalve	necrotic
capillary refill	proximal
distal	shear
hemiparesis	thrombophlebitis
ischemia	traction

1. The wound on the leg had to be debrided because it contained _____ tissue.

2. The elbow is considered _____ to the wrist.

3. The patient complained of severe pain in his foot 10 hours after the cast was applied to the ankle and the cast had to

   be _____ to relieve the pressure.

4. A cast that is too tight can cause _____ of the underlying and distal tissue.

5. The patient with a leg in traction is unable to ambulate and is at risk of _____.

6. After a cast is applied to the wrist, the nurse checks the circulation by assessing _____

   _____ of the fingers.

© 1994 W.B. Saunders Company. *Rambo's Nursing Skills for Clinical Practice,* fourth edition   289
All rights reserved.

7. When assessing adequacy of circulation after cast or traction application, the nurse checks the _____ area of the extremity.

8. The patient with _____ from a stroke often needs the assistance of a wheelchair to move around.

9. Some skeletal fractures, such as fracture of the femur, require _____ to hold the bones in place for healing.

10. When moving a patient in the bed, the nurse must be careful to avoid _____ injuries.

II. *Fill in the blank(s) with the correct word(s) or phrase.*

1. When there is inadequate physical activity, the respiratory system suffers because _____

_____.

2. Three ways to help prevent pneumonia in the immobilized patient are:

    a. _____

    b. _____

    c. _____

3. Another factor that may compromise respirations in the patient with a fracture is _____

_____.

4. Normal activity and movement of the extremities assists circulation by causing muscle contractions that

_____.

5. One way to assess for circulatory impairment is to check both _____

_____.

6. Whenever the patient has a cast or traction applied, the nurse must assess the area distal for

_____.

7. Traction is used to maintain parts of the body in _____.

© 1994 W.B. Saunders Company. *Rambo's Nursing Skills for Clinical Practice,* fourth edition
All rights reserved.

8. Potential damage from skin traction includes _____

_____ .

9. To prevent or quickly catch the occurrence of damage from skin traction, the nurse must listen to the patient and

_____ .

10. Skeletal traction makes the patient more susceptible to infection because _____

_____ .

11. Whatever type of pin care is done daily, the nurse must be especially vigilant for _____

_____ .

12. Two main aspects of nursing care for the patient in traction are to 1) keep the weights _____ ,

and the patient in _____ .

13. It is very important that the weight of traction _____ when the patient is moved
    in the bed.

14. For traction to be maximally effective, the ropes must _____ .

15. It is a great help for the immobile patient to have an _____ attached to the bed to
    assist with repositioning.

16. A possible complication for a patient freshly placed in traction with a fracture is _____

_____ caused by bone fragments.

17. Signs of this complication would include _____ and _____ .

18. To monitor for swelling, the extremity at the fracture site should be _____ upon admission.

19. While a cast is drying, it is critically important that it be protected from _____ .

20. Dents in a cast can lead to _____ and _____ .

© 1994 W.B. Saunders Company. *Rambo's Nursing Skills for Clinical Practice,* fourth edition
All rights reserved.

21. The rationale for placing a fresh cast upon pillows is that the soft, yielding, surface is less likely to _____ _____.

22. The patient with a fresh cast should be turned _____.

23. If the edges of the cast are irritating the skin, the cast can be _____ or _____.

24. When performing a cast check, always run _____ _____.

25. When the patient has a spica cast, the spreader bar must NEVER be used _____ _____.

26. Once the cast is dry and swelling has resolved, it should be checked _____ _____.

27. Walkers are helpful to patients who are _____ or who tend to _____ _____.

28. The height of the walker is correct if the person grasping the hand grips is standing upright with the elbow bent _____.

29. In order to use a walker, the person must have use of _____ _____.

30. A very important point in teaching a patient to use crutches is to teach NOT to _____ _____.

31. Crutches need to be adjusted to the individual patient both in _____ and from _____.

32. The patient is taught to walk with crutches, placing them slightly _____ _____.

© 1994 W.B. Saunders Company. *Rambo's Nursing Skills for Clinical Practice,* fourth edition
All rights reserved.

33. For proper use of a cane, the hand grip should be at hip level and the elbow should be bent _____ when weight bearing.

34. When assisting a patient into or out of a wheelchair, always _____.

35. When the wheelchair is not in motion, the _____.

36. When a patient wears a brace or prosthesis, the nurse must _____

_____ on a daily basis.

37. A major concern when transporting a patient on a stretcher is _____.

38. An air-fluidized bed is effecitve in prevention and treatment of _____ and

helps reduce _____ for the bed-fast patient.

39. Low airloss beds are contraindicated for patients with _____.

40. Continuous lateral rotation beds are used to relieve tissue pressure and to prevent or treat _____

_____.

41. Turning frames are still sometimes used for patients with _____.

42. Before turning a patient on a turning frame, be certain that _____

_____.

43. Anti-embolism stockings need to be _____ in order to be effective.

44. A very important point in nursing care for the patient wearing any type of anti-embolism stocking is to

_____ throughout the shift.

45. When using a mechanical lift, never leave the patient _____.

46. Slides and roller devices are very helpful when the nurse must _____

_____.

© 1994 W.B. Saunders Company. *Rambo's Nursing Skills for Clinical Practice,* fourth edition
All rights reserved.

47. To use a pull sheet or lift blanket, _____ are necessary.

48. A major aspect of psychosocial care for the immobilized patient is dealing with the patient's _____.

49. An immobilized patient who does not have family close by may suffer from _____ while hospitalized.

50. With the imposed inactivity that immobility causes, it is a challege to keep the patient from becoming

_____ and _____.

III. Take the post-test located at the end of the chapter in the text.

© 1994 W.B. Saunders Company. *Rambo's Nursing Skills for Clinical Practice,* fourth edition
All rights reserved.

PERFORMANCE CHECKLIST

Skill 22-1   Assessing circulation to an immobilized body part

Student: _____

Date: _____

	Satisfactory	Unsatisfactory
1. Carries out Standard Steps A, B, C, D, and E as need indicates.	❑	❑
2. Assesses pulses above and below the immobilized body part.		
a. Compares intensity of pulses and notes any discrepancy.	❑	❑
b. Lightly marks in ink the locations where pulses most easily palpated if not done by previous nurse.	❑	❑
c. Documents any pulses not accessible to palpation.	❑	❑
3. Assesses capillary refill at the distal point.		
a. Notes time interval required for color to return to normal.	❑	❑
b. Reports extension in capillary refill time (e.g. greater than 2 seconds).	❑	❑
4. Assesses sensation of distal point and compares with reported sensation on corresponding body part.	❑	❑
5. Visually assesses color of affected part and compares with color of non-affected corresponding part.	❑	❑
6. Assesses temperature of immobilized part and compares with corresponding non-affected.	❑	❑
7. Covers affected part to protect from cooling effects of exposure.	❑	❑
8. Compares all findings with those from previous assessment and notifies physician of any deterioration or developing problems.	❑	❑
9. Carries out Standard Steps X, Y, and Z.	❑	❑

Pass _____

Fail _____

Comments: _____

_____

Instructor : _____

© 1994 W.B. Saunders Company. *Rambo's Nursing Skills for Clinical Practice,* fourth edition
All rights reserved.

PERFORMANCE CHECKLIST

Skill 22-2   Skin traction care

Student: _____

Date: _____

	Satisfactory	Unsatisfactory
1. Carries out Standard Steps A, B, C, D, and E as need indicates.	❑	❑
2. Assesses leggings or wrap for presence of wrinkles or gaps.	❑	❑
3. Assesses visible skin at edges of adhesive strips for redness, swelling, lesions, or tears.	❑	❑
4. Assesses adhesive strips to see that they are firmly and uniformly attached to the skin, without bubbles or tears.	❑	❑
5. Evaluates position of extremity to see that it is in normal alignment without internal or external rotation.	❑	❑
6. Evaluates integrity of traction pull and adjusts as appropriate.	❑	❑
7. Evaluates for any potential or actual pressure against skin from mechanical parts of the traction and addresses any problems appropriately.	❑	❑
8. Carries out Standard Steps X, Y, and Z.	❑	❑

Pass _____

Fail _____

Comments: _____

_____

Instructor: _____

© 1994 W.B. Saunders Company. *Rambo's Nursing Skills for Clinical Practice,* fourth edition
All rights reserved.

PERFORMANCE CHECKLIST

Skill 22-3   Skeletal traction: Pin, tong, or wire care

Student: _____

Date: _____

		Satisfactory	Unsatisfactory
1.	Carries out Standard Steps A, B, C, D, and E as need indicates.	❏	❏
2.	Prepares all supplies for procedure using sterile technique.	❏	❏
3.	Tapes small open plastic bag to edge of table for disposal of used supplies.	❏	❏
4.	Correctly dons sterile glove.	❏	❏
5.	Cleans around pins, tongs, or wires, using a fresh swab for each site.	❏	❏
6.	Applies ointment, using fresh swab for each site.	❏	❏
7.	Carries out Standard Steps X, Y, and Z.	❏	❏

Pass _____

Fail _____

Comments: _____

_____

Instructor: _____

© 1994 W.B. Saunders Company. *Rambo's Nursing Skills for Clinical Practice,* fourth edition
All rights reserved.

PERFORMANCE CHECKLIST

Skill 22-4 Cast care

Student: _____

Date: _____

	Satisfactory	Unsatisfactory
1. Carries out Standard Steps A, B, C, D, and E as need indicates.	❑	❑
2. Examines cast for any dents.	❑	❑
3. Examines cast for areas where blood has seeped through, circles them and notes date and time. Reports excessive increase in seepage.	❑	❑
4. Checks cast for sharp edges and tightness.	❑	❑
5. Pads or covers any rough edges.	❑	❑
6. Notifies MD or cast technician of any areas which are too tight or any skin damage from rough or tight areas.	❑	❑
7. Elevates extremity with cast so hand or foot is at the level of the heart.	❑	❑
8. Places the bed in slight Trendelenburg during the first day or two for body casts, unless contraindicated by the patient's condition or physician orders.	❑	❑
9. Turns the patient at intervals so that all surfaces of the cast are exposed to air to facilitate even drying.	❑	❑
10. Instructs the patient in the dangers of using objects to scratch under the cast.	❑	❑
11. Notifies physician of severe itching and requests medication to control it.	❑	❑
12. Checks patient area for small objects that could be pushed under edges of the cast if the patient is disoriented or a young child.	❑	❑
13. Smells the open edges of the cast to assess for odor which may indicate infection under the cast.	❑	❑
14. Carries out Standard Steps X, Y, and Z.	❑	❑

Pass: _____

Fail: _____

Comments: _____

_____

Instructor: _____

© 1994 W.B. Saunders Company. *Rambo's Nursing Skills for Clinical Practice,* fourth edition
All rights reserved.

PERFORMANCE CHECKLIST

Skill 22-5   Transferring an immobile patient to a stretcher

Student: _____

Date: _____

	Satisfactory	Unsatisfactory
1. Carries out Standard Steps A, B, C, D, and E as need indicates.	❑	❑
2. Has enough staff present for safe transfer.	❑	❑
3. Prepares patient and bed for the transfer procedure, including elevating bed, locking wheels, covering patient, and removing any obstructions.	❑	❑
4. Positions any tubes so they will not be pulled or dislodged during transfer.	❑	❑
5. Performs the transfer with the assistance of other staff.		
a. Uses pull sheet.	❑	❑
b. Places stretcher firmly against open side of bed and locks wheels.	❑	❑
c. Utilizes correct body mechanics.	❑	❑
6. Fastens safety belt securely over patient and elevates stretcher side rails.	❑	❑
7. Provides for patient comfort.	❑	❑
8. Remakes or straightens bed before patient's return.	❑	❑
9. Carries out Standard Steps X, Y, and Z.	❑	❑

Pass _____

Fail _____

Comments: _____

_____

Instructor: _____

© 1994 W.B. Saunders Company. *Rambo's Nursing Skills for Clinical Practice,* fourth edition
All rights reserved.

PERFORMANCE CHECKLIST

Skill 22-6   Using a slide or roller device to transfer a Patient

Student: _____

Date: _____

	Satisfactory	Unsatisfactory
1. Carries out Standard Steps A, B, C, D, and E as need indicates.	❏	❏
2. Obtains adequate help for prevention of patient and personal injury.	❏	❏
3. Prepares patient and bed for the transfer procedure, including elevating bed, locking wheels, covering patient, and removing any obstructions.	❏	❏
4. Pulls patient toward open side of bed using pull sheet with the assistance of other staff, leaving appropriate space for roller or slide.	❏	❏
5. Places stretcher firmly against open side of bed and locks wheels.	❏	❏
6. Places the roller device on the bed between the patient and the stretcher, or places slide so it bridges the edge of the bed and the stretcher.	❏	❏
7. Moves the patient over the slide or roller using the pull sheet with assistance of other staff to the center of the stretcher.	❏	❏
8. Fastens safety belt securely over patient and elevates stretcher side rails.	❏	❏
9. Provides for patient's comfort.	❏	❏
10. Remakes or straightens patient bed before patient's return.	❏	❏
11. Carries out Standard Steps X, Y, and Z.	❏	❏

Pass _____

Fail _____

Comments: _____

_____

Instructor: _____

© 1994 W.B. Saunders Company. *Rambo's Nursing Skills for Clinical Practice,* fourth edition
All rights reserved.

PERFORMANCE CHECKLIST

Skill 22-7   Assisting a patient to transfer to a wheelchair

Student: _____

Date: _____

	Satisfactory	Unsatisfactory
1. Carries out Standard Steps A, B, C, D, and E as need indicates.	❑	❑
2. Positions the wheelchair appropriately, locks wheels and raises foot rests.	❑	❑
3. Assists patient to sit at side of bed using correct body mechanics.	❑	❑
4. Assists patient with robe and slippers.	❑	❑
5. Assists patient to stand, pivot, and sit, using correct body mechanics including a helper if needed.	❑	❑
6. Provides for patient safety while sitting up.	❑	❑
7. Encourages patient to remain sitting for a period of time to improve strength and tolerance.	❑	❑
8. Returns patient to bed after appropriate interval to prevent overtiring.	❑	❑
9. Carries out Standard Steps X, Y, and Z.	❑	❑

Pass _____

Fail _____

Comments: _____

_____

Instructor: _____

© 1994 W.B. Saunders Company. *Rambo's Nursing Skills for Clinical Practice,* fourth edition
All rights reserved.

PERFORMANCE CHECKLIST

Skill 22-8   Using a Mechanical Lift

Student: _____

Date: _____

	Satisfactory	Unsatisfactory
1. Carries out Standard Steps A, B, C, D, and E as need indicates.	❏	❏
2. Obtains another nurse to assist.	❏	❏
3. Positions chair or wheelchair as necessary and clears away any obstructions.	❏	❏
4. Elevates bed and locks wheels.	❏	❏
5. Correctly places the lift sling under the patient with the assistance of the other nurse.	❏	❏
6. Widens the stance of the lift base and locks into place.	❏	❏
7. Positions the lift correctly over the bed.	❏	❏
8. Lowers the sling hooks in a controlled manner and attaches to the sling.	❏	❏
9. Assures that all tubes are positioned so they will not be pulled or dislodged during transfer.	❏	❏
10. Asks or assists the patient to fold arms over chest.	❏	❏
11. Safely elevates the patient and moves to destination with assistance of other nurse.	❏	❏
12. Safely lowers patient into place.	❏	❏
13. Provides verbal reassurance to the patient throughout the procedure.	❏	❏
14. Positions patient in good alignment.	❏	❏
15. Covers patient, places jacket restraint if needed, and places call light within reach.	❏	❏
16. Monitors the patient at least every 15 minutes for sitting tolerance.	❏	❏
17. Maintains visual contact with any patient unable to effectively use call light.	❏	❏
18. Returns patient to bed using lift as before, following all safety precautions.	❏	❏
19. Carries out Standard Steps X, Y, and Z.	❏	❏

Pass _____

Fail _____

Comments: _____

_____

Instructor: _____

© 1994 W.B. Saunders Company. *Rambo's Nursing Skills for Clinical Practice*, fourth edition
All rights reserved.

PERFORMANCE CHECKLIST

Skill 22-9   Assisting a patient with a walker

Student: _____

Date: _____

	Satisfactory	Unsatisfactory
1. Carries out Standard Steps A, B, C, D, and E as need indicates.	❏	❏
2. Places bed in low position, lowers side rail, and assists the patient to a sitting position using correct body mechanics.	❏	❏
3. Prepares patient for ambulation.	❏	❏
4. Demonstrates the use of the walker.	❏	❏
5. Assists patient to stand and grasp hand grips on walker.	❏	❏
6. Assesses walker for correct height for patient and adjusts if necessary.	❏	❏
7. Assures that the patient is standing securely before beginning instruction.	❏	❏
8. Instructs patient in correct use of walker.	❏	❏
9. Protects patient from falling during ambulation.	❏	❏
10. Avoids overtiring the patient.	❏	❏
11. Carries out Standard Steps X, Y, and Z.	❏	❏

Pass _____

Fail _____

Comments: _____

_____

Instructor: _____

© 1994 W.B. Saunders Company. *Rambo's Nursing Skills for Clinical Practice,* fourth edition
All rights reserved.

PERFORMANCE CHECKLIST

Skill 22-10   Assisting a patient with crutches

Student: _____

Date: _____

	Satisfactory	Unsatisfactory
1. Carries out Standard Steps A, B, C, D, and E as need indicates.	❑	❑
2. Measures and adjusts the crutches to the proper length.	❑	❑
3. Prepares patient for ambulation with crutches.	❑	❑
4. Demonstrates the crutch-walking gait the patient is to use.	❑	❑
5. Assists the patient to stand with the crutches and rechecks length of the crutches with patient standing, adjusting as necessary.	❑	❑
6. Assures patient is able to maintain steady balance while standing with the crutches and only continues the training if this is so.	❑	❑
7. Instructs the patient throughout ambulation training and provides verbal encouragement and positive reinforcement.	❑	❑
8. Protects the patient from falling during ambulation.	❑	❑
9. Keeps training sessions short so patient is not overtired.	❑	❑
10. Carries out Standard Steps X, Y, and Z.	❑	❑

Pass _____

Fail _____

Comments: _____

_____

Instructor: _____

© 1994 W.B. Saunders Company. *Rambo's Nursing Skills for Clinical Practice,* fourth edition
All rights reserved.

PERFORMANCE CHECKLIST

Skill 22-11   Assisting the patient with a cane

Student: _____

Date: _____

	Satisfactory	Unsatisfactory
1. Carries out Standard Steps A, B, C, D, and E as need indicates.	❏	❏
2. Demonstrates the use of a cane for the patient.	❏	❏
3. Assists patient to stand and fastens gait belt around patient if being used.	❏	❏
4. Has patient grasp cane handle with the appropriate hand.	❏	❏
5. Instructs the patient in ambulating with a cane and provides verbal encouragement and reinforcement.	❏	❏
6. Protects patient from falling during ambulation.	❏	❏
7. Avoids overtiring the patient.	❏	❏
8. Carries out Standard Steps X, Y, and Z.	❏	❏

Pass _____

Fail _____

Comments: _____

_____

Instructor: _____

© 1994 W.B. Saunders Company. *Rambo's Nursing Skills for Clinical Practice,* fourth edition
All rights reserved.

PERFORMANCE CHECKLIST

Skill 22-12   Turning a patient in a turning frame

Student: _____

Date: _____

	Satisfactory	Unsatisfactory
1. Carries out Standard Steps A, B, C, D, and E as need indicates.	❏	❏
2. Obtains second nurse to assist with procedure.	❏	❏
3. Explains procedure to patient and verbally communicates with patient throughout procedure.	❏	❏
4. Prepares the anterior frame for use.	❏	❏
5. Removes the top covers and restraint or safety strap and assures that patient's gown covers body.	❏	❏
6. Correctly attaches the anterior frame in place over the patient and applies safety belts.	❏	❏
7. Positions all tubes so they will not be tugged or dislodged during turning of frame.	❏	❏
8. Turns patient to a prone position with assistance of second nurse.	❏	❏
9. Checks that safety locks are secure.	❏	❏
10. Removes the posterior frame.	❏	❏
11. Checks patient's alignment and adjusts as necessary.	❏	❏
12. Replaces restraint or safety strap around patient.	❏	❏
13. Carries out Standard Steps X, Y, and Z.	❏	❏

Pass _____

Fail _____

Comments: _____

_____

Instructor: _____

© 1994 W.B. Saunders Company. *Rambo's Nursing Skills for Clinical Practice,* fourth edition
All rights reserved.

PERFORMANCE CHECKLIST

Skill 22-13 Use of anti-embolism stockings

Student: _____

Date: _____

	Satisfactory	Unsatisfactory
1. Carries out Standard Steps A, B, C, D, and E as need indicates.	❏	❏
2. Measures the patient for stockings and obtains stockings of correct size.	❏	❏
3. If pulsating stockings are ordered, inserts the inflating bladders into the pockets on the sides of the stockings.	❏	❏
4. Applies the stockings, observes for correct fit, and assures there are no wrinkles or areas where the stocking bunches and binds.	❏	❏
5. Attaches tubings to bladders of pulsating stockings and observes machine for correct function.	❏	❏
6. Instructs patient not to cross legs or ankles when sitting in bed or chair.	❏	❏
7. Removes stockings at intervals as ordered, and checks for wrinkles and binding several times each shift.	❏	❏
8. Carries out Standard Steps X, Y, and Z.	❏	❏

Pass _____

Fail _____

Comments: _____

_____

Instructor: _____

© 1994 W.B. Saunders Company. *Rambo's Nursing Skills for Clinical Practice,* fourth edition
All rights reserved.

Suggested Clinical Activities

1. Actively seek assignment to patients with problems of immobility so that experience is gained in caring for patients with casts, traction, prostheses, paralysis, etc.

2. Whenever there is a special bed in use on the unit, ask the staff nurse to explain its use and any special nursing care or problems associated with the bed's use.

3. Observe a physical therapist when adjusting crutches for a patient and when teaching crutch walking.

4. Practice transfering a person with hemiparesis into and out of a wheelchair safely and smoothly. Have a peer role play the patient.

5. Ask a staff nurse to teach you to use a mechanical lift if one is available on your unit.

6. Anytime someone asks for help in transfering a patient to or from a stretcher, if possible, go and assist so that you learn all the tricks of performing this procedure efficiently and safely. Observe exactly where a slide or roller board is placed or how a lift sheet is utilized.

7. Review the instructions in the unit procedure manual for measuring the patient for application of anti-embolism stockings. Review the application of the stockings and the related nursing care, noting just how they are to be positioned on the patient, when they may be removed, how long they may remain off the patient, and how to clean them.

© 1994 W.B. Saunders Company. *Rambo's Nursing Skills for Clinical Practice,* fourth edition
All rights reserved.

Chapter 23

Fluid Balance: Intake and Output

LEARNING ACTIVITIES

I. *Vocabulary: Fill in the blank in the sentence with the correct vocabulary word.*

Vocabulary

anuria	edema
ascites	hypovolemia
dehydration	hypokalemia
diaphoresis	oliguria
diruetic	turgor

1. Mr. Thomas has no urine output and the doctor suspects his _____ is due to kidney disease.

2. When a patient's ankles are very swollen, the nurse charts that _____ of the ankles is present.

3. The medication usually prescribed for edema is a _____.

4. A young man involved in an auto accident sustained a severe cut to his leg and lost a lot of blood; he is suffering from _____.

5. An infant who has been vomiting and has diarrhea is at risk of _____.

6. After surgery, many patients suffer from _____ which a body response to the stress of surgery and the anesthesia.

7. A patient's lab work show a low potassium value. This patient has _____.

8. The abdominal swelling of the patient is caused by liver disease and is because he has _____.

9. Whenever dehydration is suspected, the patient's skin _____ is assessed.

10. Patients with high fevers often loose water due to _____.

II. Fill in the blank(s) with the correct word(s) or phrase.

1. The four ways in which fluid is lost from the body include:

   a. _____

   b. _____

   c. _____

   d. _____

2. The elderly are at risk for fluid deficit when fluid intake is decreased or a loss occurs because they have

   _____.

3. An infant is at risk for fluid deficit when fluid intake is decreased or a fluid loss occurs because it has

   _____.

4. Another reason it is important to keep track of fluid intake and output in patients who are ill is that when fluid

   balance is upset, _____ is also upset.

5. The four major electrolytes important to body function are:

   a. _____

   b. _____

   c. _____

   d. _____

6. A fluid excess is often accompanied by the electrolyte excess called _____.

7. When sodium balance shifts, the potassium balance usually shifts _____.

8. A frequent side effect of diuretic therapy is _____.

9. Signs that a fluid overload, hypervolemia, is occurring include _____

   _____.

© 1994 W.B. Saunders Company. *Rambo's Nursing Skills for Clinical Practice,* fourth edition
All rights reserved.

10. Even if a person has no fluid intake for a day, the fluid loss will amount to _____.

11. If a patient cannot take in sufficient fluids orally to maintain fluid balance, then he is given fluids _____

_____ or by _____.

12. When dehydration occurs the body compensates by _____, decreased urine output.

13. Symptoms of fluid in the peritoneal cavity, _____, include _____

_____.

14. Signs of fluid overload, fluid excess, include _____

_____.

15. Two types of patients who must be closely watched for signs of fluid excess are those with _____

_____ and _____.

III. Calculate the IV fluid intake of the patient in the following situation.

There was 280 mL remaining in the IV hanging when you came on duty at 7:00 a.m. At 9:30 you hung another IV of 1000 mL. At 3:00 p.m. there are 350 mL left in the IV bag. The total IV intake of the patient was _____ mL.

IV. Take the post-test included at the end of the chapter in the text.

© 1994 W.B. Saunders Company. *Rambo's Nursing Skills for Clinical Practice,* fourth edition
All rights reserved.

PERFORMANCE CHECKLIST

Skill 23-1   Intake and output procedure

Student: _____

Date: _____

	Satisfactory	Unsatisfactory
1. Explains procedure and gives instructions to patient about recording I & O.	❏	❏
2. Provides container for collecting urine and places measuring container in bathroom.	❏	❏
3. Records fluid intake throughout the shift.	❏	❏
4. Measures and records output throughout the shift.	❏	❏
5. At end of shift, empties collection containers, measures output and records it.	❏	❏
6. Cleans or replaces collection containers.	❏	❏
7. Calculates IV intake and records it.	❏	❏
8. Calculates total intake and total output for shift.	❏	❏
9. Enters amounts in correct columns on 24 hour I and O record.	❏	❏
10. Determines if I & O are within normal limits.	❏	❏
11. Compares amounts from previous two or three days to determine if a fluid imbalance is developing.	❏	❏
12. Places new I & O shift recording sheet in room.	❏	❏

Pass   _____

Fail   _____

Comments: _____

_____

Instructor: _____

© 1994 W.B. Saunders Company. *Rambo's Nursing Skills for Clinical Practice,* fourth edition
All rights reserved.

Suggested Clinical Activities

1. Make a list of the food and drink containers used by the dietary department in your facility and the amounts each holds.

2. Practice calculating intake for each patient assigned whether the patient is on Intake and Output recording or not.

3. Practice calculating the IV intake for each patient assigned who has an IV for the hours you are in clinical.

4. For each assigned patient, figure out what you would need to calculate for output if it was being recorded.

5. Assess each assigned patient for signs of hypokalemia.

6. Scan each assigned patient's lab values for abnormalities of electrolytes.

© 1994 W.B. Saunders Company. *Rambo's Nursing Skills for Clinical Practice,* fourth edition
All rights reserved.

Chapter 24

Diets for Varying Needs

LEARNING ACTIVITIES

I. Short answer questions.

1. Compare your weight with the recommended weight for your sex and height. Is it within the weight range, above it, or below it?

2. Compute the daily number of calories you need in order to maintain your present weight. a. Convert your weight from pounds to kilograms by dividing by 2.2 lbs per kg. b. Multiply your weight in kilograms by 24 (24 = 1 calorie per hour times the number of hours in the day.) c. Your basic caloric need for life processes is _____.

3. Now figure your total daily caloric need by multiplying the basic caloric amount by the percentage for your activity level and add the two figures. Total caloric need is_____ calories.

4. How many calories are needed to gain one pound of body weight? _____

5. The metabolic rate increases with a fever. If you have a temperature of 101 degrees F. (38.33 C.), by what percentage should your total calories increase in order to maintain your current weight? _____

6. Assume that your lunch consisted of the following foods and that you ate it all. How many calories did you consume?

    Cheese sandwich:
      Bread (2 slices)   _____
    Margarine (1 pat)   _____
    Cheese (1 ounce)   _____
    Coke (12 ounces)   _____
    Apple (1 small)   _____
       Total   _____

7. Your patient, Mrs. Weakly, has a poor appetite. With much encouragement, she ate the following for breakfast. Approximately how many calories did she get?

    Toast with butter, 2 bites (about 1/8 of a slice)   _____
    Orange juice, half of 4 oz. glass   _____
    Egg, soft-boiled, 2 bites (about 1/4 of egg)   _____
       Total   _____

II. Fill in the blank(s) with the correct word(s) or phrase.

1. Protein, a major building block, of tissue, is digested into _____ which are absorbed into the blood stream.

2. There are _____ amino acids that the body cannot produce from other sources; these are called the "essential" amino acids.

3. Food containing "complete" proteins are found in the _____ and _____ food groups.

4. The adult requirement for protein is between _____ depending on age and sex.

5. Carbohydrates are the chief _____ for the body.

6. Metabolism reduces carbohydrates to _____ which is easily transported and utilized by the body for energy.

7. Extra glucose is converted to _____ by the _____ so that it can be stored as an energy source.

8. A very important role of fats in the body is that of _____.

9. Saturated faty acids are found in _____.

10. There are also two saturated vegetable fats, _____ and _____.

11. The three essential fatty acids are necessary for the production of _____, healthy _____, _____ function, and _____ maintenance.

12. Fats provide a more concentrated form of energy for the body and provide _____ KCal per gram.

13. The fat soluble vitamins are _____, and are only absorbed when fat is present along with them in the intestinal system.

14. Vitamins are essential to the body for the _____ and proper _____.

15. Vitamin C is very important to _____.

16. The B vitamins are essential for many cellular functions, and are especially important for _____ function.

© 1994 W.B. Saunders Company. *Rambo's Nursing Skills for Clinical Practice,* fourth edition
All rights reserved.

17. Minerals are necessary for proper _____ and _____ function.

18. Generally, sufficient minerals are supplied by _____.

19. The mineral deficiency that many women develop is _____.

20. A patient needs to take in water in an amount equal to _____ plus _____.

III. Record your dietary intake for 2 days. Review your listing and calculate the number of servings per day for each of the food sets. Compare your servings with the recommended daily servings listed in the food pyramid. Are you eating a balanced diet?

IV. Take the post-test included at the end of the chapter in the text.

© 1994 W.B. Saunders Company. *Rambo's Nursing Skills for Clinical Practice,* fourth edition
All rights reserved.

PERFORMANCE CHECKLIST

Skill 24-1   Performing a basic nutritional assessment

Student: _____

Date: _____

	Satisfactory	**Unsatisfactory**
1. Carries out Standard Steps A, B, C, D, and E as need indicates.	❏	❏
2. Establishes rapport with the patient.	❏	❏
3. Utilizes nutritional assessment questions or tool to obtain data.	❏	❏
4. Determines if nutritional problem is present by analyzing the data obtained.	❏	❏
5. Documents findings and conclusions and makes nutritional referrals as needed.	❏	❏

Pass _____

Fail _____

Comments: _____

_____

Instructor: _____

© 1994 W.B. Saunders Company. *Rambo's Nursing Skills for Clinical Practice,* fourth edition
All rights reserved.

PERFORMANCE CHECKLIST

Skill 24-2   Assisting with feeding a patient

Student: _____

Date: _____

	Satisfactory	Unsatisfactory
1. Carries out Standard Steps A, B, C, D, and E as need indicates.	❑	❑
2. Checks diet tray for correct diet.	❑	❑
3. Positions the patient and the tray correctly.	❑	❑
4. Protects that patient's clothing and the bedding.	❑	❑
5. Opens the containers and prepares the food for eating.	❑	❑
6. Asks patient about preferences for order of eating foods.	❑	❑
7. Feeds slowly and without impatience.	❑	❑
8. Offers fluids as patient desires.	❑	❑
9. Wipes mouth at intervals.	❑	❑
10. Encourages patient who is able to self-feed a few bites.	❑	❑
11. Removes tray when meal is finished.	❑	❑
12. Offers mouth care and hand washing if needed.	❑	❑
13. Explains how to feed a patient who is blind or how to set up the tray and plate and to instruct the patient who is self-feeding.	❑	❑
14. Documents amount and types of food eaten.	❑	❑
15. Carries out Standard Steps X, Y, and Z.	❑	❑

Pass _____

Fail _____

Comments: _____

_____

Instructor: _____

© 1994 W.B. Saunders Company. *Rambo's Nursing Skills for Clinical Practice,* fourth edition
All rights reserved.

Suggested Clinical Activities

1. Find and look through the diet manual for the clinical facility to which you are assigned.

2. Inquire, and write down, how to notify the dietary about problems with patient trays.

3. Help a patient on a 1 gram sodium diet to choose a day's menus.

4. Review the foods that are allowed on a full liquid diet.

© 1994 W.B. Saunders Company. *Rambo's Nursing Skills for Clinical Practice,* fourth edition
All rights reserved.

Chapter 25

Nasogastric and Intestinal Tubes and Enteral Feeding

LEARNING ACTIVITIES

I. *Vocabulary: Fill in the sentences with the appropriate vocabulary word.*

     Vocabulary

decompression	gavage
distention	ileus
emesis	lavage
flatus	suction

1. Patients who cannot take in food orally are often fed by NG tube with _____ feedings.

2. After surgery, the patient who is started on feedings too quickly sometimes develops an _____.

3. An NG tube is often used during and after surgery to prevent _____.

4. After surgery on the stomach or intestine, a tube is inserted to prevent _____ of the stomach.

5. A rectal tube may be used to evacuate _____.

6. A patient who has ingested a toxin of some sort is often treated by gastric _____.

7. An NG tube is most often attached to low _____ to evacuate the stomach contents.

8. An NG tube is sometimes inserted before surgery for stomach _____.

II. *Fill in the blank(s) with the correct word(s) or phrase.*

  1. Four purposes of a stomach or intestinal tube are:

    a. _____

_____

All rights reserved.

b. _____

_____

c. _____

_____

d. _____

_____

2. A sump tube differs from other nasogastric tubes in that it _____

_____

_____

_____

3. A sump tube only works effectively if _____

_____

_____

_____

4. When caring for a patient with a nasogastric tube in place, the nurse should always _____

_____ before instilling anything into the tube.

5. If an NG tube appears to be clogged, the two methods for attempting to unclog the tube are:

a. _____ _____

b. _____

6. Tube feedings may be given _____ or _____.

7. The amount of a tube feeding generally ranges between _____ per feeding.

8. A daily amount of _____ of tube feeding is generally sufficient to meet the aptietn's nutritional requirements.

9. When a syringe is used to deliver a tube feeding, it should be _____.

10. A common side-effect of tube feedings is _____.

11. Tube feedings contain a high level of _____ and must be given slowly to prevent _____ and _____.

© 1994 W.B. Saunders Company. *Rambo's Nursing Skills for Clinical Practice,* fourth edition
All rights reserved.

12. When tube feedings are ordered for four or more times a day, they are usually started _____ and at a _____ rate.

13. Before beginning a tube feeding the patient should be positioned with the _____.

14. For a continuous feeding, the head of the bed should be kept _____.

15. Tube position should be checked before _____ or at _____.

16. Gastric residual is checked by _____

_____.

17. Accurate I and O records are important for the patient receiving tube feedings because _____

_____.

18. Stomach lavage is done in the following three instances:

    a. _____

    b. _____

    c. _____

19. A gastrostomy tube is preferred for long term feeding over an NG tube because _____

_____.

20. A jejunostomy tube is used for a patient who has had _____.

21. Long intestinal tubes are mainly used to _____.

22. The long intestinal tube is threaded into the intestine by _____.

23. In order to facilitate the movement of the intestinal tube, the patient is _____.

24. When an NG tube is attached to suction, the nurse should periodically check _____

_____.

25. Every patient who has a nasogastric tube in place should receive _____ at least once a shift, preferably every 2–4 hours.

© 1994 W.B. Saunders Company. *Rambo's Nursing Skills for Clinical Practice,* fourth edition
All rights reserved.

26. The NG tube should be positioned and attached to the patient so that it is not hanging _____

    _____.

27. Suction will be more effective for a nasogastric or intestinal tube if the connecting tubing does not hang

    _____.

28. After administering an intermittent tube feeding, the tube should be _____ with _____.

29. Another problem that the patient with a nasogastric tube often suffers is _____ due to dryness.

30. When not in use, the NG tube should be _____.

III. *Take the post-test included at the end of the chapter in the text.*

© 1994 W.B. Saunders Company. *Rambo's Nursing Skills for Clinical Practice,* fourth edition
All rights reserved.

PERFORMANCE CHECKLIST

Skill 25-1   Nasogastric tube insertion

Student: _____

Date: _____

	Satisfactory	**Unsatisfactory**
1. Carries out Standard Steps A, B, C, D, and E as indicated.	❏	❏
2. Positions patient with HOB at 30 - 90 degrees.	❏	❏
3. Agrees on signal to stop if patient desires.	❏	❏
4. Provides basin, tissues and water with straw for patient as appropriate.	❏	❏
5. Checks nostrils for best side to insert tube.	❏	❏
6. Measures distance to insert tube correctly.	❏	❏
7. Prepares tube for insertion.	❏	❏
8. Puts on gloves.	❏	❏
9. Inserts tube properly.	❏	❏
10. Verifies correct placement of tube.	❏	❏
11. Secures tube to patient.	❏	❏
12. Attaches tube to suction machine and sets machine as ordered.	❏	❏
13. Positions tube in most functional position.	❏	❏
14. Carries out Standard Steps X, Y, and Z.	❏	❏

Pass   _____

Fail   _____

Comments: _____

_____

Instructor: _____

© 1994 W.B. Saunders Company. *Rambo's Nursing Skills for Clinical Practice,* fourth edition
All rights reserved.

PERFORMANCE CHECKLIST

Skill 25-2   Irrigation of an intestinal tract tube

Student: _____

Date: _____

	Satisfactory	Unsatisfactory
1. Carries out Standard Steps A, B, C, D, and E as indicated.	❑	❑
2. Positions patient in semi-Fowler's position.	❑	❑
3. Puts on gloves.	❑	❑
4. Draws up 30–60 ml of irrigating solution.	❑	❑
5. Attaches syringe to gastric tube and aspirates to verify tube is in stomach.	❑	❑
6. Irrigates tube.	❑	❑
7. Reattaches tube to suction machine.	❑	❑
8. Notes irrigant amount on intake sheet.	❑	❑
9. Carries out Standard Steps X, Y, and Z.	❑	❑

Pass _____

Fail _____

Comments: _____

_____

Instructor: _____

© 1994 W.B. Saunders Company. *Rambo's Nursing Skills for Clinical Practice,* fourth edition
All rights reserved.

PERFORMANCE CHECKLIST

Skill 25-3 Assisting with insertion of a long intestinal tube.

Student: _____

Date: _____

	Satisfactory	Unsatisfactory
1. Carries out Standard Steps A, B, C, D, and E as indicated.	❏	❏
2. Offers support to the patient as physician inserts the tube and inflates the balloon.	❏	❏
3. Positions patient in right Sims' position.	❏	❏
4. Repositions patient per orders.	❏	❏
5. When tube reaches desired point, secures tube to patient.	❏	❏
6. Monitors suction and drainage.	❏	❏
7. Carries out Standard Steps X, Y, and Z.	❏	❏

Pass _____

Fail _____

Comments: _____

_____

Instructor: _____

© 1994 W.B. Saunders Company. *Rambo's Nursing Skills for Clinical Practice,* fourth edition
All rights reserved.

PERFORMANCE CHECKLIST

Skill 25-4 Giving an intermittent or continuous tube feeding.

Student: _____

Date: _____

	Satisfactory	Unsatisfactory
1. Carries out Standard Steps A, B, C, D, and E as indicated.	❏	❏
2. Elevates HOB 30–90 degrees.	❏	❏
3. Puts on gloves.	❏	❏
4. Prepares feeding.	❏	❏
5. Attaches syringe and verifies tube placement.	❏	❏
6. Checks for residual feeding.	❏	❏
7. Pinches off tube and pours formula into syringe or hooks up gavage bag; regulates flow correctly.	❏ ❏	❏ ❏
8. Prevents air from entering the tube.	❏	❏
9. For continuous feeding: sets up feeding pump and sets rate correctly.	❏	❏
10. Follows formula with 1–2 ounces of water to clear the tube.	❏	❏
11. Removes syringe or connecting tubing and clamps the tube for intermittent feeding.	❏	❏
12. Washes equipment appropriately.	❏	❏
13. Removes gloves	❏	❏
14. Carries out Standard Steps X, Y, and Z.	❏	❏

Pass: _____

Fail: _____

Comments: _____

_____

Instructor: _____

© 1994 W.B. Saunders Company. *Rambo's Nursing Skills for Clinical Practice,* fourth edition
All rights reserved.

PERFORMANCE CHECKLIST

Skill 25-5   Collection of a gastric specimen

Student: _____

Date: _____

	Satisfactory	**Unsatisfactory**
1. Carries out Standard Steps A, B, C, D, and E as indicated.	❏	❏
2. Positions patient in High Fowler's or sitting position.	❏	❏
3. Places the basin and tissues close to the patient.	❏	❏
4. Puts on gloves.	❏	❏
5. Measures the distance for tube insertion correctly.	❏	❏
6. Inserts tube into best nare.	❏	❏
7. Verifies tube placement and aspirates specimen.	❏	❏
8. Places specimen in labeled specimen container.	❏	❏
9. Removes tube when specimens have been collected.	❏	❏
10. Carries out Standard Steps X, Y, and Z.	❏	❏

Pass _____

Fail _____

Comments: _____

_____

Instructor: _____

© 1994 W.B. Saunders Company. *Rambo's Nursing Skills for Clinical Practice,* fourth edition
All rights reserved.

PERFORMANCE CHECKLIST

Skill 25-6   Gastric lavage

Student: _____

Date: _____

	Satisfactory	Unsatisfactory
1. Carries out Standard Steps A, B, C, D, and E as indicated.	❑	❑
2. Positions patient in Semi-Fowler's position and drapes appropriately.	❑	❑
3. Puts on gloves.	❑	❑
4. Lubricates large bore tube and inserts via the patient's mouth.	❑	❑
5. Draws out stomach contents.	❑	❑
6. Attaches syringe or funnel to tube and instills lavage solution.	❑	❑
7. Syphons out fluid; repeats process as necessary.	❑	❑
8. Pinches off tube and removes it quickly.	❑	❑
9. Carries out Standard Steps X, Y, and Z.	❑	❑

Pass _____

Fail _____

Comments: _____

_____

Instructor: _____

© 1994 W.B. Saunders Company. *Rambo's Nursing Skills for Clinical Practice,* fourth edition
All rights reserved.

PERFORMANCE CHECKLIST

Skill 25-7   Emptying or replacing the suction drainage container

Student: _____

Date: _____

		Satisfactory	Unsatisfactory
1.	Carries out Standard Steps A, B, C, D, and E as indicated.	❏	❏
2.	Turns off suction machine.	❏	❏
3.	Puts on gloves.	❏	❏
4.	Removes stopper from drainage container or canister from the machine.	❏	❏
5.	Uses protective eyewear when measuring and disposing of drainage.	❏	❏
6.	Cleans and reinstalls container.	❏	❏
7.	Removes gloves and discards appropriately.	❏	❏
8.	Reinstitutes suction as ordered.	❏	❏
9.	Verifies suction system is functioning.	❏	❏
10.	Carries out Standard Steps X, Y, and Z.	❏	❏

Pass _____

Fail _____

Comments: _____

_____

Instructor: _____

© 1994 W.B. Saunders Company. *Rambo's Nursing Skills for Clinical Practice,* fourth edition
All rights reserved.

PERFORMANCE CHECKLIST

Skill 25-8   Removal of gastrointestinal tract tubes

Student: _____

Date: _____

	Satisfactory	**Unsatisfactory**
1. Carries out Standard Steps A, B, C, D, and E as indicated.	❏	❏
2. Untapes the tube.	❏	❏
3. Puts on gloves.	❏	❏
4. Positions towel or basin to receive tube.	❏	❏
5. Pinches off tube and removes gently but quickly.	❏	❏
6. Disposes of tube.	❏	❏
7. Offers mouth care.	❏	❏
8. Measures and records gastric drainage; cleans or replaces drainage container.	❏	❏
9. Removes gloves and discards correctly.	❏	❏
10. Carries out Standard Steps X, Y, and Z.	❏	❏

Pass _____

Fail _____

Comments: _____

_____

Instructor: _____

© 1994 W.B. Saunders Company. *Rambo's Nursing Skills for Clinical Practice,* fourth edition
All rights reserved.

Suggested Clinical Activities

1. Ask a staff nurse to show you how to prepare a feeding pump and institute a continuous tube feeding.

2. Survey the staff nurses on your unit and find out their suggestions for dealing with a clogged feeding tube. Are their suggestions "safe"?

3. Perform an assessment on a patient receiving tube feedings to determine the degree of benefit the patient is receiving.

4. Interview five patients who have a nasogastric tube. What are their complaints? What can be done to make them more comfortable?

© 1994 W.B. Saunders Company. *Rambo's Nursing Skills for Clinical Practice,* fourth edition
All rights reserved.

Chapter 26

Urinary Care and Catheterization

LEARNING ACTIVITIES

I. Vocabulary. Fill in the appropriate word to complete the sentence.

Vocabulary

cystitis	irrigation
diuresis	meatus
incontinence	void

1. Approximately 48 hours after surgery and anesthesia, the patient usually experiences _____, and the urine output increases.

2. Symptoms of _____ include urgency, and pain upon urination.

3. When performing a male catheterization, it is necessary to clean the urinary _____.

4. When the nurse needs a urine specimen the patient is asked to _____ into a specimen container.

5. The patient who cannot control the urinary sphincter experiences urinary _____.

6. After a transurethral resection of the prostate, the patient usually has a continuous bladder _____

   _____ set-up.

II. Fill in the blank(s) with the correct word(s) or phrase.

1. If the bladder is not emptied urine will build up back-pressure and cause _____.

2. Urinary bladder control is usually achieved by about age _____.

3. A tube inserted into the kidney itself to drain urine or pus is called a _____ tube.

All rights reserved.

4. Bladder instillations using medication are done for treatment of _____.

5. When the kidneys cease to function sufficiently to remove waste products from the blood it is necessary to perform

_____.

6. Normal urine is usually a shade of _____.

7. The lighter the color of urine, the more _____ it is.

8. An unpleasant odor from urine may indicate _____.

9. The normal specific gravity of urine is _____.

10. The normal pH of urine is _____.

11. A fracture pan is used when _____.

12. When placing a fracture pan, the wide lip goes _____.

13. At least _____ of urine is needed for a routine urinalysis.

14. For a mid-stream urine specimen, the patient is first asked to _____

_____.

15. While obtaining a mid-stream specimen, the patient should begin voiding and _____

_____.

16. For a 24 hour urine specimen collection, the patient's bladder should be _____ at the beginning and at the end of the collection.

17. Urine specimens should be transported to the laboratory promptly because _____

_____.

18. Organisms most commonly found to cause bladder infections include _____

_____.

© 1994 W.B. Saunders Company. *Rambo's Nursing Skills for Clinical Practice,* fourth edition
All rights reserved.

19. It is very important that any catheter inserted into the urinary bladder be inserted using _____.

20. When catheterizing a female, it is wise to identify the location of _____ before opening the catheter kit.

21. All patients who have an indwelling urinary catheter are placed on _____ recording.

22. With a closed drainage system, it is important to keep the drainage container _____ _____.

23. When a retention catheter is removed, it is essential that the _____ first.

24. After the retention catheter is removed, the patient must void normally within _____.

25. A problem that many patients with indwelling catheters experience in the hospital is _____ _____.

26. Suprapubic catheters are often used after gynecologic surgery so that _____ can be re-established before the catheter is removed.

27. Bladder irrigations must be done maintaining strict _____.

28. When performing a bladder irrigation, the nurse must be careful not to exert _____ _____.

29. Continuous ambulatory peritoneal dialysis allows the patient to _____ _____.

30. For each peritoneal dialysis treatment, approximately _____ of dialysate solution is instilled.

31. The return solution after peritoneal dialysis should be _____.

32. A frequent complication of peritoneal dialysis is _____ and can be prevented by the use of _____.

© 1994 W.B. Saunders Company. *Rambo's Nursing Skills for Clinical Practice,* fourth edition
All rights reserved.

33. When caring for a peritoneal dialysis patient, the nurse must assess for _____ and for

_____.

34. Prior to the peritoneal dialysis treatment, the patient's vital signs are taken and the patient is _____

_____.

35. Accurate _____ records are essential for the patient receiving peritoneal dialysis.

III. *Take the post-test included at the end of the chapter in the text.*

© 1994 W.B. Saunders Company. *Rambo's Nursing Skills for Clinical Practice,* fourth edition
All rights reserved.

PERFORMANCE CHECKLIST

Skill 26-1 Using the bedpan

Student: _____

Date: _____

	Satisfactory	Unsatisfactory
1. Carries out Standard Steps A, B, C, D, and E as need indicates.	❑	❑
2. Correctly places bedpan under the patient and positions patient.	❑	❑
3. Provides tissue and call light.	❑	❑
4. Removes the bedpan without spilling the contents.	❑	❑
5. Assists the patient to cleanse the perineal area if needed.	❑	❑
6. Measures and records the urine output.	❑	❑
7. Cleans the equipment.	❑	❑
8. Allows patient to wash the hands.	❑	❑
9. Removes gloves and washes own hands.	❑	❑
10. Carries out Standard Steps X, Y, and Z.	❑	❑

Pass _____

Fail _____

Comments: _____

_____

Instructor: _____

© 1994 W.B. Saunders Company. *Rambo's Nursing Skills for Clinical Practice,* fourth edition
All rights reserved.

PERFORMANCE CHECKLIST

Skill 26-2   Assisting with a urinal

Student: _____

Date: _____

	Satisfactory	**Unsatisfactory**
1. Carries out Standard Steps A, B, C, D, and E as need indicates.	❑	❑
2. Gives urinal to patient or assists with positioning.	❑	❑
3. Provides privacy; and places call light at hand.	❑	❑
4. Removes urinal, measures and discards urine.	❑	❑
5. Allows patient to wash his hands.	❑	❑
6. Cleanses the urinal.	❑	❑
7. Washes own hands.	❑	❑
8. Carries out Standard Steps X, Y, and Z.	❑	❑

Pass _____

Fail _____

Comments: _____

_____

Instructor: _____

© 1994 W.B. Saunders Company. *Rambo's Nursing Skills for Clinical Practice,* fourth edition
All rights reserved.

PERFORMANCE CHECKLIST

Skill 26-3   Testing for glucose and acetone in the urine

Student: _____

Date: _____

		Satisfactory	Unsatisfactory
1.	Carries out Standard Steps A, B, C, D, and E as need indicates.	❑	❑
2.	Reads directions for test ordered.	❑	❑
3.	Obtains fresh urine specimen.	❑	❑
4.	Performs test correctly.	❑	❑
5.	Records results accurately.	❑	❑
6.	Cleans equipment.	❑	❑
7.	Carries out Standard Steps X, Y, and Z.	❑	❑

Pass _____

Fail _____

Comments: _____

_____

Instructor: _____

© 1994 W.B. Saunders Company. *Rambo's Nursing Skills for Clinical Practice,* fourth edition
All rights reserved.

PERFORMANCE CHECKLIST

Skill 26-4 Female straight catheterization

Student: _____

Date: _____

	Satisfactory	Unsatisfactory
1. Carries out Standard Steps A, B, C, D, and E as indicated.	❑	❑
2. Opens catheter tray and positions it appropriately while maintaining sterile technique.	❑	❑
3. Dons sterile gloves correctly.	❑	❑
4. Holds labia open throughout cleaning and catheterization.	❑	❑
5. Cleanses the perineal area correctly, stroking front to back; uses forceps to hold the cotton balls.	❑	❑
6. Lubricates and inserts catheter correctly, maintaining sterility.	❑	❑
7. Drains the urine from the bladder and removes the catheter.	❑	❑
8. Cleans up equipment and the patient.	❑	❑
9. Measures and records amount of urine.	❑	❑
10. Carries out Standard Steps X, Y, and Z.	❑	❑

Pass _____

Fail _____

Comments: _____

_____

Instructor: _____

© 1994 W.B. Saunders Company. *Rambo's Nursing Skills for Clinical Practice,* fourth edition
All rights reserved.

PERFORMANCE CHECKLIST

Skill 26-5   Male straight catheterization

Student: _____

Date: _____

	Satisfactory	**Unsatisfactory**
1. Carries out Standard Steps A, B, C, D, and E as need indicates.	❏	❏
2. Opens the catheter tray and sets up work area maintaining a sterile field.	❏	❏
3. Dons gloves correctly.	❏	❏
4. Prepares specimen container if needed.	❏	❏
5. Cleanses the penis and meatal opening with antiseptic swabs, using forceps.	❏	❏
6. Lubricates the catheter and correctly inserts it into the bladder.	❏	❏
7. Collects a urine specimen if required.	❏	❏
8. Finishes draining the urine from the bladder.	❏	❏
9. Removes the catheter without dribbling urine.	❏	❏
10. Prepares and labels the specimen if one was obtained.	❏	❏
11. Carries out Standard Steps X, Y, and Z.	❏	❏

Pass _____

Fail _____

Comments: _____

_____

Instructor: _____

© 1994 W.B. Saunders Company. *Rambo's Nursing Skills for Clinical Practice,* fourth edition
All rights reserved.

PERFORMANCE CHECKLIST

Skill 26-6   Insertion of a retention (Foley) catheter

Student: _____

Date: _____

		Satisfactory	**Unsatisfactory**
1.	Carries out Standard Steps A, B, C, D, and E as need indicates.	❏	❏
2.	Opens catheter kit and arranges sterile field maintaining sterility.	❏	❏
3.	Dons sterile gloves correctly.	❏	❏
4.	Tests balloon on catheter and deflates it.	❏	❏
5.	Cleanses area correctly with forceps, antiseptic solution and cotton balls.	❏	❏
6.	Lubricates and inserts catheter maintaining sterility.	❏	❏
7.	Inflates balloon, positions catheter correctly.	❏	❏
8.	Cleans up used supplies and cleans and dries perineal area of patient.	❏	❏
9.	Hangs drainage bag correctly and positions tubing to promote best drainage.	❏	❏
10.	Secures catheter to the patient.	❏	❏
11.	Carries out Standard Steps X, Y, and Z.	❏	❏

Pass _____

Fail _____

Comments: _____

_____

Instructor: _____

© 1994 W.B. Saunders Company. *Rambo's Nursing Skills for Clinical Practice,* fourth edition
All rights reserved.

PERFORMANCE CHECKLIST

Skill 26-7   Removal of a retention catheter

Student: _____

Date: _____

	Satisfactory	**Unsatisfactory**
1. Carries out Standard Steps A, B, C, D, and E as indicated.	❏	❏
2. Checks volume of balloon; removes tape or leg band securing catheter.	❏	❏
3. Inserts the empty syringe into the balloon stem valve and withdraws all water.	❏	❏
4. Pinches off the catheter and removes the catheter gently; catches catheter in paper towel.	❏	❏
5. Empty drainage bag and measure the urine; record the output.	❏	❏
6. Carries out Standard Steps X, Y, and Z.	❏	❏

Pass _____

Fail _____

Comments: _____

_____

Instructor: _____

© 1994 W.B. Saunders Company. *Rambo's Nursing Skills for Clinical Practice,* fourth edition
All rights reserved.

PERFORMANCE CHECKLIST

Skill 26-8   Application of a condom catheter

Student: _____

Date: _____

	Satisfactory	**Unsatisfactory**
1. Carries out Standard Steps A, B, C, D, and E as indicated.	❏	❏
2. Washes and dries genital area; trims pubic hair as necessary.	❏	❏
3. Applies condom catheter and smooths out adhesive surface for good adherence.	❏	❏
4. Leaves a 1-1/2 in. space at tip of penis.	❏	❏
5. Connects the condom catheter to a drainage tube.	❏	❏
6. Attaches drainage bag.	❏	❏
7. Checks to see that catheter has not become twisted, preventing urine flow.	❏	❏
8. Carries out Standard Steps X, Y, and Z.	❏	❏

Pass _____

Fail _____

Comments: _____

_____

Instructor: _____

© 1994 W.B. Saunders Company. *Rambo's Nursing Skills for Clinical Practice,* fourth edition
All rights reserved.

PERFORMANCE CHECKLIST

Skill 26-9 Suprapubic catheter care

Student: _____

Date: _____

	Satisfactory	Unsatisfactory
1. Carries out Standard Steps A, B, C, D, and E as indicated.	❏	❏
2. Checks catheter for patency q shift.	❏	❏
3. Maintains sterility of closed drainage system.	❏	❏
4. Monitors for signs of urinary tract infection.	❏	❏
5. Replaces dressing at insertion site prn; cleanses area before applying dressing.	❏	❏
6. Clamps catheter as ordered and monitors patient comfort.	❏	❏
7. Has patient void and checks for residual.	❏	❏
8. Performs patient teaching for home self-care.	❏	❏
9. Documents appropriately,	❏	❏
10. Carries out Standard Steps X, Y, and Z.	❏	❏

Pass _____

Fail _____

Comments: _____

_____

Instructor: _____

© 1994 W.B. Saunders Company. *Rambo's Nursing Skills for Clinical Practice,* fourth edition
All rights reserved.

PERFORMANCE CHECKLIST

Skill 26-10　Bladder irrigation

Student: _____

Date: _____

	Satisfactory	Unsatisfactory
1. Carries out Standard Steps A, B, C, D, and E as indicated.	❏	❏
2. Opens irrigation tray and sets up sterile field without contaminating equipment.	❏	❏
3. Pours irrigation solution.	❏	❏
4. Dons gloves.	❏	❏
5. Clamps connecting tubing or disconnects tubing from catheter, maintaining aseptic technique.	❏	❏
6. Draws up solution and instills it into the catheter either directly or via the injection port.	❏	❏
7. Uses 30–50 cc of solution for each irrigation.	❏	❏
8. Allows the irrigation fluid to flow back.	❏	❏
9. Continues to irrigate 3 - 4 times.	❏	❏
10. Withdraws syringe, wipes catheter and tube connections with fresh antiseptic swab and reconnects tubing.	❏	❏

FOR CONTINUOUS IRRIGATION

	Satisfactory	Unsatisfactory
11. Sets up Murphy drip for continuous bladder irrigation and regulates it as ordered.	❏	❏
12. Assesses system for patency and function q 30 min.	❏	❏
11. Carries out Standard Steps X, Y, and Z.	❏	❏

Pass _____

Fail _____

Comments: _____

_____

Instructor: _____

© 1994 W.B. Saunders Company. *Rambo's Nursing Skills for Clinical Practice,* fourth edition
All rights reserved.

PERFORMANCE CHECKLIST

Skill 26-11   Obtaining a urine specimen from a retention catheter and closed drainage system.

Student: _____

Date: _____

	Satisfactory	Unsatisfactory
1. Carries out Standard Steps A, B, C, D, and E as indicated.	❏	❏
2. Prepares sterile specimen container.	❏	❏
3. Clamps the catheter for twenty minutes.	❏	❏
4. Swabs injection port with fresh antiseptic swab.	❏	❏
5. Inserts needle with syringe and withdraws 5–10 ml of urine.	❏	❏
6. Places urine in specimen container.	❏	❏
7. Disposes of needle and syringe in sharps container.	❏	❏
8. Unclamps catheter.	❏	❏
9. Labels specimen and sends it to the laboratory.	❏	❏
10. Carries out Standard Steps X, Y, and Z.	❏	❏

Pass _____

Fail _____

Comments: _____

_____

Instructor: _____

© 1994 W.B. Saunders Company. *Rambo's Nursing Skills for Clinical Practice,* fourth edition
All rights reserved.

PERFORMANCE CHECKLIST

Skill 26-12   Peritoneal dialysis care

Student: _____

Date: _____

	Satisfactory	Unsatisfactory
1. Carries out Standard Steps A, B, C, D, and E as indicated.	❏	❏
2. Obtains baseline weight and vital signs.	❏	❏
3. Warms dialysate solution.	❏	❏
4. Injects medications, if ordered.	❏	❏
5. Cleans connection on Tenchoff catheter and connects tubing.	❏	❏
6. Opens clamp and slowly runs in dialysate solution; monitors the patient.	❏	❏
7. Clamps the tubing for designated dwell time.	❏	❏
8. Lowers the bags or bottles and unclamps the tubing for return drainage.	❏	❏
9. Repeats the process as ordered.	❏	❏
10. Records data on flow sheet, keeping accurate I & O.	❏	❏
11. Inspects return fluid for signs of abnormality.	❏	❏
12. Provides general nursing care during the procedure.	❏	❏
13. Carries out Standard Steps X, Y, and Z.	❏	❏

Pass _____

Fail _____

Comments: _____

_____

Instructor: _____

© 1994 W.B. Saunders Company. *Rambo's Nursing Skills for Clinical Practice,* fourth edition
All rights reserved.

Suggested Clinical Activities

1. Practice catheterization procedure until you can do it efficiently and aseptically five times in the skill lab. Have a peer evaluate you as you do the procedure.

2. Ask to observe catheterization procedures on your assigned unit before attempting to perform one.

3. With a peer, practice comfortably placing a bedpan under a patient. Use water to partially fill the pan and practice removing it without spilling "urine".

4. If possible, observe a nurse as she performs peritoneal dialysis for a patient.

5. Practice obtaining a sterile specimen from the retention catheter set-up in the skill lab.

6. Practice removing a retention catheter in the skill lab.

7. Accompany another nurse to observe when a retention catheter is to be removed.

© 1994 W.B. Saunders Company. *Rambo's Nursing Skills for Clinical Practice,* fourth edition
All rights reserved.

Chapter 27

Bowel Elimination

LEARNING ACTIVITIES

I. Fill in the blank(s) with the correct word(s) or phrase.

1. List the three functions of the digestive system.

    a. _____

    b. _____

    c. _____

2. The accessory digestive organs include the _____, _____, and _____.

3. Partially digested food mixed with enzymes is called _____.

4. _____ is the term used to describe the muscular activity of the intestinal tract.

5. The _____, _____, and _____ make up the small intestine.

6. Absorption of _____ and _____ occurs in the small intestine.

7. List the two main functions of the large intestines. _____

    _____

    _____

8. _____ is an excessive amount of bleeding.

9. _____ is a liquid or semiliquid stool.

10. _____ is a dilated blood vessel around the anus.

11. State four of the problems related to the function of elimination.

   a. _____

   b. _____

   c. _____

   d. _____

12. The long length of the intestinal tract and the circular folds within the tract provide a greater surface for

   _____ to take place.

13. The various parts of the intestinal tract have been described. In the following list, indicate the parts of the large intestine.

   a. ileum _____

   b. rectum _____

   c. colon _____

   d. jejunum _____

   e. cecum _____

   f. duodenum _____

   g. anus _____

14. Feces consist of one-fourth _____ and three-fourths _____.

15. The color of the normal stool is _____.

16. One of your patients, Mr. Long, has just had a bowel movement that is black in appearance and tarry in consistency.

   This means that the stool contains _____, which probably came from the (duodenum) (cecum)

   (sigmoid colon). (Circle one.)

17. Hemorrhage in the large intestine produces a stool characterized by _____.

18. Pale, clay-colored stools are due to the absence of _____.

19. A slick, slimy appearance of the stool is caused by _____.

20. The rapid movement of chyme in the hyperactive bowel interferes with _____ and
   results in _____.

© 1994 W.B. Saunders Company. *Rambo's Nursing Skills for Clinical Practice,* fourth edition
All rights reserved.

21. _____ is caused by a hypoactive bowel.

22. Purposes for using rectal suppositories are

a. _____

b. _____ or

c. _____

23. When placed correctly, the rectal suppository

a. stimulates the outer surface of the rectum.
b. is in contact with the inner surface of the rectum.
c. melts inside the fecal mass in the rectum.
d. lies between the anal sphincter and the anal rectal ridges.

For a cleansing enema given to an adult, indicate the specific information in connection with the following:

24. Kind of solution used _____

25. Amount of solution _____

26. Temperature of the solution _____

27. Height of the solution container above the anus _____

28. State at least two possibe reasons for the patient to have difficulty during the administration of an enema.

a. _____

b. _____

29. The inability of a person to control their bowels is called _____.

30. List the three ways a person can maintain regular bowel elimination and the three initial steps in a bowel retraining program.

a. _____

b. _____

c. _____

31. _____, _____, and _____ are medications which may be used as a part of a bowel retraining program.

II. Take the post-test included at the end of the chapter in the text.

© 1994 W.B. Saunders Company. *Rambo's Nursing Skills for Clinical Practice*, fourth edition
All rights reserved.

PERFORMANCE CHECKLIST

Skill 27-1 Collection of a stool specimen

Student: _____

Date: _____

	Satisfactory	**Unsatisfactory**
1. Carries out Standard Steps A, B, C, D, and E as need indicates.	❑	❑
2. Requests that patient save next stool and notify desk when specimen is available.	❑	❑
3. Dons gloves and prepares specimen properly and transfers it to the specimen container.	❑	❑
4. Places lid on container, cleans equipment and disposes of soiled tongue blades and gloves.	❑	❑
5. Labels specimen container and completes the laboratory request slip; sends specimen to the laboratory expediently.	❑	❑
6. Carries out Standard Steps X, Y, and Z.	❑	❑

Pass _____

Fail _____

Comments: _____

_____

Instructor: _____

© 1994 W.B. Saunders Company. *Rambo's Nursing Skills for Clinical Practice,* fourth edition
All rights reserved.

PERFORMANCE CHECKLIST

Skill 27-2   Performing a stool guaiac test

Student: _____

Date: _____

	Satisfactory	Unsatisfactory
1. Carries out Standard Steps A, B, C, D and E as need indicates.	❑	❑
2. Obtains an appropriate stool specimen.	❑	❑
3. Dons gloves and prepares sample of stool for testing.	❑	❑
4. Adds reagent and times test accurately.	❑	❑
5. Correctly reads test result.	❑	❑
6. Carries out Standard Steps X, Y, and Z.	❑	❑

Pass _____

Fail _____

Comments: _____

_____

Instructor: _____

© 1994 W.B. Saunders Company. *Rambo's Nursing Skills for Clinical Practice,* fourth edition
All rights reserved.

PERFORMANCE CHECKLIST

Skill 27-3 Inserting a rectal suppository

Student: _____

Date: _____

	Satisfactory	**Unsatisfactory**
1. Carries out Standard Steps A, B, C, D, and E as need indicates.	❑	❑
2. Positions patient correctly.	❑	❑
3. Dons gloves; removes wrapper and lubricates suppository.	❑	❑
4. Inserts suppository.	❑	❑
5. Carries out Standard Steps X, Y, and Z.	❑	❑

Pass _____

Fail _____

Comments: _____

_____

Instructor: _____

© 1994 W.B. Saunders Company. *Rambo's Nursing Skills for Clinical Practice,* fourth edition
All rights reserved.

PERFORMANCE CHECKLIST

Skill 27-4   Administering various types of enemas

Student: _____

Date: _____

	Satisfactory	Unsatisfactory
1. Carries out Standard Steps A, B, C, D, and E as need indicates.	❏	❏
2. Positions the patient appropriately.	❏	❏
3. Prepares the enema, clears air from tubing, and lubricates tip.	❏	❏
4. Positions bedpan or bedside commode; places under- pad beneath patient.	❏	❏
5. Dons gloves and gently inserts the rectal tip correct distance.	❏	❏
6. Positions fluid no higher than 18" or squeezes plastic bottle to instill the solution.	❏	❏
7. Regulates flow according to patient's amount of discomfort.	❏	❏
8. Clamps tubing before withdrawing the tip.	❏	❏
9. Assists patient onto bedpan, bedside commode, or to toilet.	❏	❏
10. Instills correct amount of solution for total enema.	❏	❏
11. Assists patient to clean anal area if needed.	❏	❏
12. Carries out Standard Steps X, Y, and Z.	❏	❏

Pass _____

Fail _____

Comments: _____

_____

Instructor: _____

© 1994 W.B. Saunders Company. *Rambo's Nursing Skills for Clinical Practice,* fourth edition
All rights reserved.

PERFORMANCE CHECKLIST

Skill 27-5   Administering a Harris flush enema

Student: _____

Date: _____

	Satisfactory	**Unsatisfactory**
1. Carries out Standard Steps A, B, C, D, and E as need indicates.	❑	❑
2. Positions patient appropriately.	❑	❑
3. Prepares solution.	❑	❑
4. Dons gloves, lubricates tip and gently inserts tubing tip into anus the correct distance.	❑	❑
5. Holds solution no higher than 18 inches.	❑	❑
6. Lowers container at least 12 inches below the anus and allows solution to flow back.	❑	❑
7. Repeats the in and out flow of solution 4–5 times.	❑	❑
8. Carries out Standard Steps X, Y, and Z.	❑	❑

Pass _____

Fail _____

Comments: _____

_____

Instructor: _____

© 1994 W.B. Saunders Company. *Rambo's Nursing Skills for Clinical Practice,* fourth edition
All rights reserved.

PERFORMANCE CHECKLIST

Skill 27-6   Removal of a fecal impaction

Student: _____

Date: _____

		Satisfactory	**Unsatisfactory**
1.	Carries out Standard Steps A, B, C, D, and E as need indicates.	❏	❏
2.	Dons gloves and arranges the bedpan and toilet tissue on a chair by the bed; lubricates the index finger well.	❏	❏
3.	Inserts lubricated finger into the rectum, and gently dislodges or breaks up stool and removes it piece by piece.	❏	❏
4.	Removes all stool within reach.	❏	❏
5.	Carries out Standard Steps X, Y, and Z.	❏	❏

Pass _____

Fail _____

Comments: _____

_____

Instructor: _____

© 1994 W.B. Saunders Company. *Rambo's Nursing Skills for Clinical Practice,* fourth edition
All rights reserved.

Suggested Clinical Activities

1. With a peer to observe technique, practice giving an enema to a mannequin in the skill lab. Practice until you are comfortable with the equipment and the procedure.

2. Work with a patient or relative who has a long-standing problem with constipation on a bowel retraining program.

3. Ask on the assigned unit for an opportunity to obtain and test a stool specimen for occult blood.

4. Seek clinical opportunities to give an enema.

© 1994 W.B. Saunders Company. *Rambo's Nursing Skills for Clinical Practice,* fourth edition
All rights reserved.

Chapter 28

Ostomy Care

LEARNING ACTIVITIES

I. Fill in the blank(s) with the correct word(s) or phrase.

1. Many patients who have a new ostomy are also dealing with the problems of _____ as well.

2. Patients facing an ostomy frequently experience _____
   _____.

3. An ostomy procedure causes a major change in the person's _____ and a readjustment of life-style.

4. When a patient is in denial about the need for an ostomy, a meeting with a professional _____
   _____ or _____ nurse therapist is suggested.

5. It is important that the stoma site chosen for the ostomy be _____ by the patient to facilitate self-care.

6. A valuable resource for the ostomy patient is the _____.

7. The three general types of ostomies are the:

   a. _____

   b. _____

   c. _____

8. A continent diversion is emptied by _____.

9. An advantage of a continent diversion is that the patient does not have to _____
   _____.

All rights reserved.

10. The patient who has an ileostomy is at risk for the complication of _____

_____.

11. Drainage from a ureteral stent should be _____.

12. The patient with a continent diversion will return from surgery with a _____ in place.

13. The stoma should be _____ or _____ in appearance.

14. A stoma that is _____ or _____ must be reported immediately.

15. Complications of an ostomy procedure include _____

_____.

16. The new ostomy patient undergoes considerable emotional stress and will take time to adjust _____ _____ to the stoma and situation.

17. The new ostomy patient has many teaching needs, of which _____ care is of prime importance.

18. If the ostomy patient has a history of skin problems or allergies, it is wise to do _____

_ _____ before apply-

ing an adhesive to the stoma site.

19. The nurse should assess _____ and _____ daily for every
post-operative ostomy patient.

20. An ultimate goal for the ostomy patient is total _____.

II. *Take the post-test included at the end of the chapter in the text.*

© 1994 W.B. Saunders Company. *Rambo's Nursing Skills for Clinical Practice,* fourth edition
All rights reserved.

PERFORMANCE CHECKLIST

Skill 28-1   Colostomy irrigation

Student: _____

Date: _____

	Satisfactory	Unsatisfactory
1. Carries out Standard Steps A, B, C, D, and E as need indicates.	❑	❑
2. Washes hands and dons gloves.	❑	❑
3. Explains procedure to patient.	❑	❑
4. Assists patient as needed to assume comfortable position on toilet or commode, or side-lying in bed if bedfast.	❑	❑
5. Removes old pouch and disposes of correctly.	❑	❑
6. Cleanses and dries skin and stoma, observing condition and color.	❑	❑
7. Applies and secures irrigating sleeve.	❑	❑
8. Fills irrigation container with warm water and hangs at correct level.	❑	❑
9. Flushes air from tubing.	❑	❑
10. Inserts catheter tip into stoma and seats cone.	❑	❑
11. Begins water flow slowly, increasing rate based on patient tolerance.	❑	❑
12. If water does not flow, repositions tube and assures there are no kinks in tubing to obstruct flow.	❑	❑
13. Allows remainder of water to flow in at steady, moderate rate, slowing or discontinuing if patient is unable to retain.	❑	❑
14. Removes catheter, closes hole in top of irrigation sleeve, and allows adequate time for bowel evacuation.	❑	❑
15. Rinses the sleeve with water, rolls the end closed and secures it when most of the stool has been expelled.	❑	❑
16. When evacuation complete, removes and rinses irrigation sleeve and hangs to dry.	❑	❑
17. Cleanses skin, applies clean pouch and skin barriers as appropriate, trimming opening as needed.	❑	❑
18. Assists patient back to bed as necessary.	❑	❑
19. Carries out Standard Steps X, Y, and Z.	❑	❑

Pass _____

Fail _____

Comments: _____

_____

Instructor: _____

© 1994 W.B. Saunders Company. *Rambo's Nursing Skills for Clinical Practice,* fourth edition
All rights reserved.

PERFORMANCE CHECKLIST

Skill 28-2 Application of new ostomy pouch

Student: _____

Date: _____

	Satisfactory	Unsatisfactory
1. Carries out Standard Steps A, B, C, D, and E as need indicates.	❑	❑
2. Washes hands and dons gloves.	❑	❑
3. Prepares pouch wafer.	❑	❑
4. Empties and removes old pouch and disposes of properly.	❑	❑
5. Cleanses skin with warm water or pre-moistened towelette.	❑	❑
6. Applies skin barrier and pouch.	❑	❑
7. Apples tape around skin barrier edges and attaches belt if indicated.	❑	❑
8. Carries out Standard Steps X, Y, and Z.	❑	❑

Pass _____

Fail _____

Comments: _____

_____

Instructor: _____

© 1994 W.B. Saunders Company. *Rambo's Nursing Skills for Clinical Practice,* fourth edition
All rights reserved.

Suggested Clinical Activities

1. Contact an enterostomal therapist, if available, and ask to go along on some patient visits and teaching sessions.

2. Attend the local Ostomy society meeting.

3. Obtain a copy of the literature available for ostomy patients from the local chapter of the American Cancer Society.

4. In the clinical setting, seek an opportunity to observe a colostomy irrigation, ileostomy care, and urostomy care.

© 1994 W.B. Saunders Company. *Rambo's Nursing Skills for Clinical Practice,* fourth edition
All rights reserved.

Chapter 29

Using Surgical Asepsis

LEARNING ACTIVITIES

I. Vocabulary. Fill in the sentence with the appropriate word from the vocabulary list.

> *Vocabulary*
>
> contaminated   purulent
> disinfect   surgical asepsis
> germocide   virulence
> pathogen

1. Both surgical asepsis and medical asepsis are used to prevent the transmission of a _____ from one item or person to another.

2. After a surgical suite is used, it is treated with a _____ to decrease the number of microorganisms present.

3. If the nurse turns so that the sterile field is out of the visual field, the field is considered _____.

4. When a wound becomes infected it is often _____.

5. Keeping an area free from microorganisms is done by practicing _____.

6. The magnitude of the disease process is dependent on the _____ of the pathogen involved.

7. Disinfection of furniture and permanent items in a room is usually done by application of a _____.

II. Fill in the blank(s) with the correct word(s) or phrase.

1. The goal of surgical asepsis is to _____.

2. The first line of defense against infection is provided by _____.

© 1994 W.B. Saunders Company. *Rambo's Nursing Skills for Clinical Practice,* fourth edition 419
All rights reserved.

3. Organisms transfer to the host via the following four ways:

    a. _____

    b. _____

    c. _____

    d. _____

4. Organisms can enter the body via:

    a. _____

    b. _____

    c. _____

    d. _____

5. Organisms leave the body via:

    a. _____

    b. _____

    c. _____

    d. _____

6. The development of an infection depends on the following three factors:

    a. _____

    b. _____

    c. _____

7. The practice of surgical asepsis is directed toward preventing contamination of _____

_____ and _____.

8. A surgical scrub is a mechanical cleansing meant to _____

_____.

9. The surgical scrub covers an area from the tips of the fingers to_____.

10. _____ is the body's response to any type of injury.

© 1994 W.B. Saunders Company. *Rambo's Nursing Skills for Clinical Practice,* fourth edition
All rights reserved.

11. The five cardinal signs of inflammation are:

    a. _____

    b. _____

    c. _____

    d. _____

    e. _____

12. The four cardinal rules of asepsis are:

    a. _____

    b. _____

    c. _____

    d. _____

13. Sterile items wrapped in cloth must be resterilized every _____.

14. Contamination occurs when a sterile surface _____.

15. There are three ways to remedy the situation when contamination has occurred:

    a. _____

    b. _____

    c. _____

16. Sterile materials must be kept _____ because _____

    _____

17. Sterile fields are often contaminated by reaching _____.

18. For gloves to remain sterile while worn, they must remain _____ and above

    _____.

19. The first flap on a sterile package is opened _____.

20. When donning sterile gloves, each glove should be picked up and held in an area between _____

    _____ and about _____ from the body.

© 1994 W.B. Saunders Company. *Rambo's Nursing Skills for Clinical Practice,* fourth edition
All rights reserved.

III. Take the post-test included at the end of the chapter in the text.

© 1994 W.B. Saunders Company. *Rambo's Nursing Skills for Clinical Practice,* fourth edition
All rights reserved.

PERFORMANCE CHECKLIST

Skill 29-1   Using a disposable mask

Student: _____

Date: _____

	Satisfactory	Unsatisfactory
1. Puts on face mask before scrubbing.	❏	❏
2. Handles mask by ties or cord.	❏	❏
3. Fits mask firmly to nose and face covering both mouth and nose.	❏	❏
4. Takes off mask handling it by the ties or cord.	❏	❏
5. Disposes of mask properly.	❏	❏

Pass _____

Fail _____

Comments: _____

_____

Instructor: _____

© 1994 W.B. Saunders Company. *Rambo's Nursing Skills for Clinical Practice,* fourth edition
All rights reserved.

PERFORMANCE CHECKLIST

Skill 29-2   Performing a surgical hand scrub

Student: _____

Date: _____

	Satisfactory	Unsatisfactory
1. Removes jewelry.	❑	❑
2. Adjusts water to correct temperature and force.	❑	❑
3. Wets hands and arms from above elbows to fingertips, keeping hands higher than elbows.	❑	❑
4. Applies soaping agent or uses soap impregnated brush or sponge pad. Works up a lather.	❑	❑
5. Cleans nails on each hand while holding the scrub brush/pad in other hand.	❑	❑
6. Starts scrubbing at fingertips with a circular motion scrubs each finger, between fingers, palm and back of hand using light to moderate friction; scrubs wrist and up the arm to 2" above the elbow.	❑	❑
7. Scrubs each arm for approximately 2–2 1/2 minutes. Times the scrub by the clock.	❑	❑
8. Rinses each hand and arm thoroughly keeping the hands pointed up and allowing water to run from the fingertips down off of the elbow area.	❑	❑
9. Disposes of brush/pad by dropping it into the proper receptacle.	❑	❑
10. Turns off water using foot or knee control.	❑	❑
11. Dries hands with a sterile towel without contaminating sterile field or scrubbed hands.	❑	❑
12. Drops used towel into proper receptacle.	❑	❑

Pass _____

Fail _____

Comments: _____

_____

Instructor: _____

© 1994 W.B. Saunders Company. *Rambo's Nursing Skills for Clinical Practice,* fourth edition
All rights reserved.

PERFORMANCE CHECKLIST

Skill 29-3   Opening sterile packs and preparing a sterile field

Student: _____

Date: _____

	Satisfactory	**Unsatisfactory**
1. Carries out Standard Steps A, B, C, D, and E as indicated for the procedure.	❏	❏
2. Clears a working surface.	❏	❏
3. Removes outer wrap.	❏	❏
4. Opens pack with proper aseptic technique.	❏	❏
5. Arranges items on the sterile field.	❏	❏
6. Performs procedure.	❏	❏
7. Carries out Standard Steps X, Y, and Z.	❏	❏

Pass _____

Fail _____

Comments: _____

_____

Instructor: _____

© 1994 W.B. Saunders Company. *Rambo's Nursing Skills for Clinical Practice,* fourth edition
All rights reserved.

PERFORMANCE CHECKLIST

Skill 29-4   Opening and using individually wrapped sterile supplies

Student: _____

Date: _____

	Satisfactory	**Unsatisfactory**
1. Peels the package apart at the proper location in a downward motion.	❏	❏
2. Offers the sterile item to another person.	❏	❏
3. Demonstrates how to open the package flat on a clean surface.	❏	❏
4. Demonstrates how to drop a sterile item onto a sterile field.	❏	❏
5. Disposes of package wrappers.	❏	❏

Pass _____

Fail _____

Comments: _____

_____

Instructor: _____

© 1994 W.B. Saunders Company. *Rambo's Nursing Skills for Clinical Practice,* fourth edition
All rights reserved.

PERFORMANCE CHECKLIST

Skill 29-5   Using sterile transfer forceps

Student: _____

Date: _____

	Satisfactory	Unsatisfactory
1. Establishes a dry, sterile field.	❑	❑
2. Opens package of sterile forceps correctly; or obtains sterile forceps from container.	❑	❑
3. Opens the forceps keeping the tips pointed down.	❑	❑
4. Grasps the sterile article and transfers it over the sterile field and drops it in the desired location.	❑	❑
5. Positions forceps with handles off the sterile field.	❑	❑
6. Returns reusable forceps to the container.	❑	❑
7. Disposes of wrappers from supplies.	❑	❑

Pass _____

Fail _____

Comments: _____

_____

Instructor: _____

© 1994 W.B. Saunders Company. *Rambo's Nursing Skills for Clinical Practice,* fourth edition
All rights reserved.

PERFORMANCE CHECKLIST

Skill 29-6   Pouring a sterile liquid

Student: _____

Date: _____

	Satisfactory	Unsatisfactory
1. Verifies that the correct solution is in the bottle.	❏	❏
2. Removes bottle cap and sets it down without contaminating the lip of the bottle or the cap.	❏	❏
3. Positions receiving container appropriately for pouring within the sterile field.	❏	❏
4. Holds the bottle with the label facing self and pours from about a 6" height; does not splash onto the sterile field.	❏	❏
5. Recaps the bottle and sets it outside of the sterile field.	❏	❏

Pass _____

Fail _____

Comments: _____

_____

Instructor: _____

© 1994 W.B. Saunders Company. *Rambo's Nursing Skills for Clinical Practice,* fourth edition
All rights reserved.

PERFORMANCE CHECKLIST

Skill 29-7 Sterile gloving and ungloving

Student: _____

Date: _____

	Satisfactory	**Unsatisfactory**
1. Obtains pair of sterile gloves of correct size; washes hands.	❏	❏
2. Peels open outer wrapper and positions inner glove package on flat surface.	❏	❏
3. Opens the inner glove package exposing the gloves without contaminating them.	❏	❏
4. Picks up the first glove by the folded over cuff.	❏	❏
5. Inserts hand into glove without touching the outside of the glove to any part of the skin or other unsterile object; keeps hands above waist level.	❏	❏
6. Picks up the second glove by placing gloved fingers under the cuff; slips hand into the glove being careful not to allow bare skin to touch the other gloved hand.	❏	❏
7. Slides cuffs over the wrists; adjusts the fingers inside the gloves.	❏	❏

UNGLOVING

	Satisfactory	Unsatisfactory
8. Grasps the outside surface of one glove at the top of the palm and pulls glove off while rolling it inside out.	❏	❏
9. Holds removed glove in palm of other hand; slips bare fingers under the cuff of the remaining glove and slides the glove down over the hand, rolling it inside-out as it is removed.	❏	❏
10. Disposes of the contaminated gloves.	❏	❏
11. Washes the hands.	❏	❏

Pass _____

Fail _____

Comments: _____

_____

Instructor: _____

© 1994 W.B. Saunders Company. *Rambo's Nursing Skills for Clinical Practice,* fourth edition
All rights reserved.

Suggested Clinical Activities

1. Practice the surgical scrub in the skill lab, or home simulated situation, until you are comfortable with the procedure. Have a peer observe your technique.

2. Seek assignment to areas where surgical asepsis is mandatory, i.e., the O.R., Emergency Room, Labor and Delivery, the Nursery.

3. Go with other nurses to observe the way in which they set up a sterile field for a dressing change or treatment.

4. Practice setting up a sterile field and opening sterile packages in the skill lab if possible. Have a peer observe your technique.

5. Observe for breaks in asepsis when working with other nurses; decide how you would have avoided the break and how to remedy it.

© 1994 W.B. Saunders Company. *Rambo's Nursing Skills for Clinical Practice*, fourth edition
All rights reserved.

Chapter 30

Preoperative Care

LEARNING ACTIVITIES

I. Vocabulary. Fill in the sentence with the appropriate word from the vocabulary list.

Vocabulary	Suffixes
anesthesia	-cele
aspirate	-ectomy
cyanosis	-oma
hemorrhage	-ostomy
laparotomy	-plasty
NPO	

1. Whenever a patient is to have surgery involving a general anesthetic, his orders will read "_____ after midnight".

2. The reason that patients receive nothing by mouth for 8 - 12 hours before surgery is so they don't _____ during or right after surgery.

3. A _____ is performed to inspect the abdominal organs in a patient who has sustained abdominal trauma and is experiencing complications.

4. _____ of the skin indicates that the patient is not getting sufficient oxygen circulated to the tissues.

5. _____ for surgery can be partial or complete depending on whether the patient is undergoing a major or minor surgical procedure.

6. A rectocele is a _____ of the rectum.

7. An appendectomy is the _____ of the appendix.

8. An adenoma is a _____ of a gland.

9. A colostomy is an _____ into the colon.

All rights reserved.

10. A rhinoplasty is a _____ of the nose.

11. A _____ may occur internally or externally.

II. Fill in the blank(s) with the correct word(s) or phrase.

1. The three major goals of the nurse in preparing the patient for surgery are:

   a. _____

   b. _____

   c. _____

2. If an abnormality in vital signs occurs the morning of surgery, the surgery may need to be _____.

3. Maintaining the NPO status of the patient is primarily to prevent _____ in reaction to anesthesia.

4. When a patient is NPO, the nurse should indicate that _____ is also prohibited.

5. If the patient does eat or drink anything while on NPO status, the surgery will need to be _____.

6. Patients need to be reminded that the only clothing to be worn to surgery is _____ and the nurse should check again that no underwear is in place as the patient leaves the unit.

7. Before surgery, medications are usually given to _____.

8. The purpose of skin preparation prior to surgery is to _____

   _____.

9. Whenever a patient leaves the unit for surgery, all orders are _____.

10. The same day or ambulatory surgery patient has a great need for _____ as well as physical preparation.

11. Successful healing without complications for the same day or ambulatory surgery patient is greatly dependent upon

    good _____.

© 1994 W.B. Saunders Company. *Rambo's Nursing Skills for Clinical Practice,* fourth edition
All rights reserved.

12. Paper work to be completed before the patient goes to surgery includes a _____

    and a preoperative _____.

13. Generally, lab work required before surgery includes both a _____ and a _____.

14. After surgery, the patient is taken to the Post Anesthesia Care Unit where vital signs are checked every

    _____.

15. Patients at increased risk for complications during or after surgery include: (list at least 5)

    a. _____

    b. _____

    c. _____

    d. _____

    e. _____

16. An important part of a preoperative nursing assessment is checking for allergies to _____,

    _____, and _____.

17. When using clippers to prep the skin, the skin should be _____.

18. When evaluating preoperative teaching about deep breathing, the nurse should have the patient

    _____.

19. Patients often fear general anesthesia because they think they might _____.

20. When preoperative medication is ordered, the nurse must check to see that the _____
    before administering the medication.

III. *Take the post-test included at the end of the chapter in the text.*

© 1994 W.B. Saunders Company. *Rambo's Nursing Skills for Clinical Practice,* fourth edition
All rights reserved.

PERFORMANCE CHECKLIST

Skill 30-1   Surgical skin preparation with shave prep

Student: _____

Date: _____

	Satisfactory	Unsatisfactory
1. Carries out Standard Steps A, B, C, D, and E as indicated.	❏	❏
2. Works up a soapy lather.	❏	❏
3. Holds skin taut while shaving.	❏	❏
4. Strokes in same direction as hair growth.	❏	❏
5. Scrubs from center outward.	❏	❏
6. Inspects to see that all hair is removed.	❏	❏
7. Carries out Standard Steps X, Y, and Z.	❏	❏

Pass _____

Fail _____

Comments: _____

_____

Instructor: _____

© 1994 W.B. Saunders Company. *Rambo's Nursing Skills for Clinical Practice,* fourth edition
All rights reserved.

PERFORMANCE CHECKLIST

Skill 30-2 Preoperative teaching to prevent complications

Student: _____

Date: _____

	Satisfactory	Unsatisfactory
1. Carries out Standard Steps A, B, C, D, and E as indicated.	❏	❏
2. Shows patient how to turn in bed while splinting incision.	❏	❏
3. With patient in sitting position, demonstrates deep breathing technique.	❏	❏
4. Has patient practice deep breathing.	❏	❏
5. Demonstrates huff coughing technique.	❏	❏
6. Has patient practice huff coughing.	❏	❏
7. Shows patient how to do leg and foot exercises.	❏	❏
8. Has patient perform leg and foot exercises.	❏	❏
9. Carries out Standard Steps X, Y, and Z.	❏	❏

Pass _____

Fail _____

Comments: _____

_____

Instructor: _____

© 1994 W.B. Saunders Company. *Rambo's Nursing Skills for Clinical Practice,* fourth edition
All rights reserved.

PERFORMANCE CHECKLIST

Skill 30-3   Completing the preoperative checklist

Student: _____

Date: _____

	Satisfactory	Unsatisfactory
1. Carries out Standard Steps A, B, C, D, and E as indicated.	❑	❑
2. Takes equipment, chart and preoperative checklist to patient's bedside.	❑	❑
3. Verifies I.D. number and correct name on I.D. band.	❑	❑
4. Checks blood bracelets if blood was ordered.	❑	❑
5. Verifies that the chart is in order with surgical/anesthesia consent, lab and diagnostic test results, and history and physical.	❑	❑
6. Takes and records vital signs.	❑	❑
7. Has patient void and dress in hospital gown.	❑	❑
8. Secures valuables; tapes ring if worn.	❑	❑
9. Has patient remove prostheses; labels and stores prostheses appropriately.	❑	❑
10. Verifies when last food and fluids were taken.	❑	❑
11. Rechecks for allergies.	❑	❑
12. Performs preoperative head-to-toe assessment.	❑	❑
13. Administers preoperative medications efficiently.	❑	❑
14. Institutes safety precautions after preoperative medications have been given.	❑	❑
15. Completes preoperative checklist and charts documentation.	❑	❑
16. Assists with transfer of patient to stretcher and verification of patient identification.	❑	❑
17. Directs significant others to waiting area.	❑	❑
18. Prepares unit for patient's return.	❑	❑

Pass _____

Fail _____

Comments: _____

_____

Instructor: _____

© 1994 W.B. Saunders Company. *Rambo's Nursing Skills for Clinical Practice,* fourth edition
All rights reserved.

Suggested Clinical Activities

1. Make up your own preoperative assessment "checklist" and put the outline on a card you can carry with you to use until you are very familiar with the assessment routine.

2. Whenever you are assigned a preoperative patient, carefully plan the time necessary to complete the preoperative care, the preoperative medication doses, and the necessary documentation. Remember that the preoperative patient's care is a high priority.

3. Accompany other nurses when they do preoperative teaching and preoperative care and complete the checklist so that you become comfortable with the routine.

4. Seek opportunities to care for preoperative patients. Ask to be assigned to the same day surgery unit at least for a day to gain experience in giving preoperative care and preparing and giving preoperative medications.

© 1994 W.B. Saunders Company. *Rambo's Nursing Skills for Clinical Practice,* fourth edition
All rights reserved.

Chapter 31

Intraoperative Care

LEARNING ACTIVITIES

I. Fill in the blank(s) with the correct word(s) or phrase.

1. The use of heat to destroy microorganisms was promoted by _____.

2. Lister believing that disease was caused by microorganisms began the use of _____ on dressings.

3. Major surgery is defined as a surgical procedure that is _____ that can lead to

   more _____.

4. The six purposes of surgery include:

   a. _____

   b. _____

   c. _____

   d. _____

   e. _____

   f. _____

5. The introduction of _____ and _____ has made many surgical procedures less traumatic than before.

6. The staff in an O.R. where a laser is to be used must _____ in order to avoid reflected beams of laser light.

7. To maintain a minimum of bacterial growth, the operating suite is kept at _____ degrees F. and at _____ humidity.

8. Whenever it is in doubt as to whether an item is sterile, it is _____.

© 1994 W.B. Saunders Company. *Rambo's Nursing Skills for Clinical Practice,* fourth edition
All rights reserved.

9. The scrub nurse's duties include _____

_____.

10. The circulating nurse functions by _____

_____.

11. Scrub clothes are _____ not _____.

12. The surgical team wears sterile _____ and _____ plus _____,

_____, _____, and either shoe covers or special

_____.

13. When preparing and replacing instruments on the sterile field, hemostats and clamps are closed
_____.

14. For denuding the skin or hair, clippers or a depilatory are used rather than a razor because _____

_____.

15. The final skin prep in the O.R. consists of applying a _____, rinsing, and then

applying a _____.

16. The circulating nurse is considered the _____ of the operating room.

17. The _____ nurse has prime responsibility for the maintenance of sterile technique.

18. An important duty of the scrub nurse is to count _____ before the surgical
procedure begins and at the end before the incision is closed.

19. A primary duty of the circulating nurse is to see that the patient is transferred safely to the operating table and is

_____.

20. Masks should be changed between operations and whenever _____.

21. Conversation in the O.R. should be _____.

© 1994 W.B. Saunders Company. *Rambo's Nursing Skills for Clinical Practice,* fourth edition
All rights reserved.

22. Between surgical cases, a short, _____ scrub is performed.

23. When donning a sterile gown, it is necessary to have _____ assist by

   _____.

24. Proper identification of the patient for a specific surgical procedure is done by _____

   _____.

25. Verification of the surgical procedure to be performed is done by noting the entry on the _____

   _____.

II. Take the post-test included at the end of the chapter in the text.

© 1994 W.B. Saunders Company. *Rambo's Nursing Skills for Clinical Practice,* fourth edition
All rights reserved.

PERFORMANCE CHECKLIST

Skill 31-1   Modified surgical scrub

Student: _____

Date: _____

	Satisfactory	**Unsatisfactory**
1. Puts on mask and protective eyewear before beginning scrub.	❑	❑
2. Adjusts water temperature and force.	❑	❑
3. Uses soap and brush or sponge pad for scrub.	❑	❑
4. Scrubs each skin surface correct number of strokes or amount of time.	❑	❑
5. Rinses well keeping fingertips pointed up and hands above elbow level.	❑	❑
6. Picks up sterile towel without contaminating the hands.	❑	❑
7. Dries thoroughly keeping arms above waist level.	❑	❑
8. Discards towel without lowering arms below waist level.	❑	❑

Pass _____

Fail _____

Comments: _____

_____

Instructor: _____

© 1994 W.B. Saunders Company. *Rambo's Nursing Skills for Clinical Practice,* fourth edition
All rights reserved.

PERFORMANCE CHECKLIST

Skill 31-2   Self-gowning technique

Student: _____

Date: _____

	Satisfactory	Unsatisfactory
1. Picks up sterile gown without contaminating self, gown, or table.	❑	❑
2. Allows gown to unfold correctly.	❑	❑
3. Places arms into armholes and eases into gown; uses help of assistant to straighten, position, and fasten gown.	❑	❑
4. Ties waist tie without contaminating self.	❑	❑

Pass _____

Fail _____

Comments: _____

_____

Instructor: _____

© 1994 W.B. Saunders Company. *Rambo's Nursing Skills for Clinical Practice,* fourth edition
All rights reserved.

PERFORMANCE CHECKLIST

Skill 31-3   Closed surgical gloving

Student: _____

Date: _____

	Satisfactory	Unsatisfactory
1. Picks up and positions right glove without contaminating glove.	❑	❑
2. Pulls on right glove properly without contaminating the glove.	❑	❑
3. Picks up and positions left glove without contaminating either glove.	❑	❑
4. Pulls on left glove properly without contaminating either glove.	❑	❑
5. Straightens gloves for smooth fit.	❑	❑
6. Keeps hands above waist level.	❑	❑

Pass _____

Fail _____

Comments: _____

_____

Instructor: _____

© 1994 W.B. Saunders Company. *Rambo's Nursing Skills for Clinical Practice,* fourth edition
All rights reserved.

PERFORMANCE CHECKLIST

Skill 31-4 Gowning and gloving another person

Student: _____

Date: _____

	Satisfactory	**Unsatisfactory**
1. Properly hands gownee a sterile towel.	❑	❑
2. Unfolds and holds sterile gown so gownee can place arms in armholes without contaminating own gloved hands.	❑	❑
3. Has unsterile worker assist gownee with positioning and fastening the gown.	❑	❑
4. Picks up and positions right glove properly so that gownee can place the right hand in the glove; keeps glove above waist level.	❑	❑
5. Picks up and positions left glove properly so that gownee can place the left hand in the glove; keeps glove above waist level.	❑	❑

Pass _____

Fail _____

Comments: _____

_____

Instructor: _____

© 1994 W.B. Saunders Company. *Rambo's Nursing Skills for Clinical Practice,* fourth edition
All rights reserved.

PERFORMANCE CHECKLIST

Skill 31-5   Withdrawing sterile solution from a vial

Student: _____

Date: _____

	Satisfactory	Unsatisfactory
1. Obtains vial and performs check of solution or medication using the "five rights".	❑	❑
2. Verifies the vial and solution or medication with another person.	❑	❑
3. Cleanses the vial stopper with antiseptic swab.	❑	❑
4. Holds vial, label up, so that scrubbed person can insert needles and withdraw the solution.	❑	❑
5. Keeps hands above waist level.	❑	❑
6. Disposes of vial appropriately when finished.	❑	❑

Pass _____

Fail _____

Comments: _____

_____

Instructor: _____

© 1994 W.B. Saunders Company. *Rambo's Nursing Skills for Clinical Practice,* fourth edition
All rights reserved.

Suggested Clinical Activities

1. Practice sterile gowning and gloving in the skill lab if possible. Have a peer evaluate your technique.

2. Practice setting up an instrument table in the skill lab if possible. Have a peer evaluate your technique.

3. Perform a full surgical scrub and then immediately gown and glove; be certain to prepare your gown and gloves before scrubbing.

4. Ask to observe in the O.R. for a clinical day or two.

5. If assigned to the O.R., question the circulating nurse about her duties; ask her how the scrub nurse's duties are different.

6. Ask to accompany an assigned patient to surgery and observe the operation.

7. When observing in surgery, note how breaks in sterile technique are handled.

© 1994 W.B. Saunders Company. *Rambo's Nursing Skills for Clinical Practice,* fourth edition
All rights reserved.

Chapter 32

Postoperative Care

LEARNING ACTIVITIES

I. Fill in the blank(s) with the correct word(s) or phrase.

1. In the postoperative period, the effects of surgery and the anesthesia on the patient are characterized by

   a. _____ and

   b. _____

2. The functions of nursing consist of the a. _____ and b. _____ aspects.

3. Orders for the postoperative care of the patient are written by

   a. the charge nurse.
   b. the doctor.
   c. the ward clerk.
   d. the anesthesiologist.

4. As a beginning worker in nursing, where would you most likely give postoperative care to the patient?

   _____

5. When is the patient transferred from the PACU to his or her own room? _____

6. Hyperventilation should be suspected when the respirations are a. _____ and b. _____.

7. The unconscious patient should be turned every _____ hours.

8. The common obstructions of the airway are a. _____ and b. _____.

9. Why is it advisable to turn the unconscious patient's head to one side? _____

   _____

10. The underlying cause of most respiratory complications is _____.

© 1994 W.B. Saunders Company. *Rambo's Nursing Skills for Clinical Practice,* fourth edition   467
All rights reserved.

11. To increase respiratory function, you should assist and encourage the postoperative patient to

    a. _____ b. _____ , and c. _____ .

12. Two complications that result from decreased respiratory functions are a. _____ and b.

    _____ .

13. In the postoperative patient, the cause of shock is usually _____ .

14. A patient going into shock would have early signs that include a. _____ , b. _____ , and

    c. _____ .

15. When you observe signs of shock in your patient,what is the first thing you should do? _____

    _____

16. The treatment of shock by the nurse-doctor team, in which you also participate, consists of:

    a. _____

    b. _____

    c. _____

    d. _____

    e. _____

    f. _____

17. What is meant by fluid balance? _____

18. An adult who is convalescing well after surgery has a total output of 2150 ml forthe 24-hour period. What should the

    intake have been? _____

19. When is the patient expected to void following surgery? _____

20. The most common types of tubes the patient may have following surgery are

    a. _____

    b. _____ and

    c. _____

© 1994 W.B. Saunders Company. *Rambo's Nursing Skills for Clinical Practice,* fourth edition
All rights reserved.

21. To reduce the possibility of danger or harm to the patient in the first hours following surgery, you would take the following steps:

    a. _____

    b. _____

    c. _____

    d. _____

22. Which of the following statements refers to a nursing activity that provides for the patient's safety?

    a. The nurse closely observes the patient to help maintain his respiratory and circulatory functions.
    b. The nurse takes care to prevent dislodging the IV needle from the vein when turning a patient who is receiving IV fluid.
    c. After assisting the patient to use the bedpan for voiding, the nurse washes her hands before taking the patient's vital signs.
    d. Every two hours, the nurse assists and encourages the patient who has recovered from anesthesia to breathe deeply, cough, and turn.

Mrs. Lily returned from the recovery room a short time ago. You have taken the vital signs and have noted the following:

Time	BP	P	R
1115	128/78	88	20
1130	112/70	100	20
1145	108/60	112	20

23. What might this indicate to you? _____

24. What should you do now? _____

25. Mr. Willis had surgery last week and his vital signs have been within the normal ranges for several days. However, this morning his temperature was 37.6C (approximately 99.8F) at 0600. How often should you take his vital signs today? _____

26. Almost without exception, the postoperative patient will experience the discomfort of _____.

27. The depressing action of drugs and anesthesia causes hypoactivity of the bowel and contributes to the discomfors of

    a. _____ and b. _____.

© 1994 W.B. Saunders Company. *Rambo's Nursing Skills for Clinical Practice,* fourth edition
All rights reserved.

28. The patient had surgery about ten hours ago and is allowed to take fluids and diet as tolerated but continues to have moderate nausea. Some actions you might take to reduce the patient's nausea are:

   a. _____

   b. _____

   c. _____

   d. _____

   e. _____

29. Mr. Sloan had an operation on his stomach three hours ago. Which of the following conditions would lead you to suspect that he may be hemorrhaging? More than one answer may be corret.

   a. You notice more dark reddish-brown drainage on his abdominal dressing.
   b. He has started moving restlessly from side to side, his eyes seem to roll around, and he is moaning.
   c. In the last few minutes, the Levin tube has filled with bright red drainage.
   d. His IV fluids have slowed down to a rate of 20 drops per minute.
   e. His pulse is now 116 beats per minute, but had been around 60 to 80 in surgery.

30. The day after surgery, Mr. Sloan asked you to put a pillow under his knees to ease the strain on his abdomen and also

   wanted you to rub his legs because they seemed sore. What would you do and why? _____

   _____

31. Name those measures you can take to prevent thrombophlebitis from becoming a complication for Mr. Sloan.

   a. _____

   b. _____

   c. _____

32. Wound infections produce inflammation; the symptoms of inflammation are:

   a. _____

   b. _____

   c. _____

   d. _____

   e. _____

33. Evisceration means the exposure of _____.

   II. Take the post-test included at the end of the chapter in the text.

© 1994 W.B. Saunders Company. *Rambo's Nursing Skills for Clinical Practice,* fourth edition
All rights reserved.

PERFORMANCE CHECKLIST

Skill 32-1   Assessment during the immediate postoperative period

Student: _____

Date: _____

	Satisfactory	Unsatisfactory
1. Carries out Standard Steps A, B, C, D, and E as need indicates.	❏	❏
2. Transfers patient safely to the postoperative bed; moves IV solution to IV pole.	❏	❏
3. Assesses airway and respirations; starts oxygen therapy if ordered.	❏	❏
4. Checks IV to see that it is patent and at correct flow rate; adjusts flow rate if needed.	❏	❏
5. Measures vital signs per scheduled times.	❏	❏
6. Checks incisional area and dressing.	❏	❏
7. Checks each tube for function and patency.	❏	❏
8. Assesses peripheral pulses.	❏	❏
9. Assesses for pain and offers comfort measures.	❏	❏
10. Auscultates heart, lungs, and abdomen.	❏	❏
11. Offers mouth care at appropriate intervals.	❏	❏
12. Continues assessments and interventions on schedule during immediate postoperative period.	❏	❏
13. Carries out Standard Steps X, Y, and Z.	❏	❏

Pass _____

Fail _____

Comments: _____

_____

Instructor: _____

© 1994 W.B. Saunders Company. *Rambo's Nursing Skills for Clinical Practice,* fourth edition
All rights reserved.

PERFORMANCE CHECKLIST

Skill 32-2   Care of the vomiting patient

Student: _____

Date: _____

	Satisfactory	Unsatisfactory
1. Carries out Standard Steps A, B, C, D, and E as need indicates. (Wears glove.)	❏	❏
2. Moves patient slowly for repositioning.	❏	❏
3. Uses damp cloth on face and neck when patient voices nausea.	❏	❏
4. Keeps room odor free.	❏	❏
5. Instructs patient in breathing techniques to decrease nausea and prevent vomiting.	❏	❏
6. Provides emesis basin and tissues.	❏	❏
7. Cleanses patients face after vomiting and removes emesis basin.	❏	❏
8. Measures and documents amount and characteristics of vomitus.	❏	❏
9. Cleans and replaces emesis basin.	❏	❏
10. Gives mouth care.	❏	❏
11. Advances diet slowly and provides teaching.	❏	❏
12. If patient continues vomiting, obtains order for antiemetic.	❏	❏
13. Carries out Standard Steps X, Y, and Z.	❏	❏

Pass _____

Fail _____

Comments: _____

_____

Instructor: _____

© 1994 W.B. Saunders Company. *Rambo's Nursing Skills for Clinical Practice,* fourth edition
All rights reserved.

Suggested Clinical Activities

1. Accompany a nurse who is receiving a patient back from surgery to observe the immediate postoperative assessment and care.

2. Ask to be assigned to a patient who will be returning from surgery on your shift. Perform the postoperative assessment and immediate post-operative care. Remember to plan the time needed for frequent assessment and vital signs in your work schedule.

3. Assist a patient to perform postoperative breathing, coughing, and leg exercises.

4. Assess the pain management for the first 24 hours post-op for two or three patients. Would you handle the pain management differently?

5. Begin instructing the postoperative patient for self-care, considering wound care, diet, activity, elimination, rest, pain control, and medications.

© 1994 W.B. Saunders Company. *Rambo's Nursing Skills for Clinical Practice,* fourth edition
All rights reserved.

Chapter 33

Wound and Skin Care

LEARNING ACTIVITIES

I. Vocabulary. Insert the appropriate word in the sentence using the vocabulary list.

Vocabulary

abscess	exudate
adhesion	fistula
debride	infection
eschar	pressure wound
erythema	purulent

1. One sign of inflammation around a wound is _____.

2. When eschar is present, it is necessary to _____ the wound.

3. The abdominal incision is swollen, painful, reddened, and warm, indicating the probable presence of an

    _____.

4. Sometimes an _____ forms after surgery, firmly connecting two surfaces of tissue.

5. The _____ from the wound was clear and non-odorous.

6. The patient unfortunately developed a _____ between the rectum and the vagina.

7. The presence of pus in a wound indicates an _____.

8. Dark, tough tissue around or within a wound is called _____ and must be debrided.

9. An _____ wound takes longer to heal than a clean wound.

10. A _____ most frequently occurs over bony prominences.

© 1994 W.B. Saunders Company. *Rambo's Nursing Skills for Clinical Practice,* fourth edition   477
All rights reserved.

II. Fill in the blank(s) with the correct word(s) or phrase.

1. If one sign of inflammation is present, the nurse should _____

    _____.

2. One drug that can suppress or mask the signs of infection is _____.

3. A wound that involves cellular necrosis is called a _____.

4. Pressure points that should be inspected frequently include _____

    _____.

5. Pressure ulcers form when pressure on the tissue decreases _____.

6. A pressure ulcer may occur within a few hours in the _____.

7. Damage to skin already compromised by pressure can be further aggravated by _____

    _____   _____.

8. Prevention of pressure ulcers is the responsibility of _____.

9. Skin inspection on every patient should be performed at least _____.

10. Areas where pressure has occurred should be inspected when _____.

11. The patient's position must be changed at least _____.

12. Avoid side positioning where pressure is _____.

13. _____ rather than drag patients who cannot assist with repositioning.

14. Two examples of pressure reducing devices include

    a. _____

    b. _____

15. A reddened area should never be _____.

© 1994 W.B. Saunders Company. *Rambo's Nursing Skills for Clinical Practice,* fourth edition
All rights reserved.

16. An area that is reddened, intact, and does not blanch with light pressure is classed as a _____ pressure ulcer.

17. Reddening accompanied by a blister, abrasion, or shallow area of skin loss is classed as a _____ pressure ulcer.

18. A stage III pressure ulcer is an area that has _____

_____.

19. The difference between a Stage III and a Stage IV pressure ulcer is that the Stage IV pressure ulcer _____

_____.

20. A wound is considered "clean" if _____.

21. Granulation tissue appears _____.

22. A healing wound should be measured at least _____.

23. Seven factors that can adversely affect wound healing include:

    a. _____

    b. _____

    c. _____

    d. _____

    e. _____

    f. _____

    g. _____

24. Excessive growth of scar tissue over a wound site is called a _____.

25. The best way to prevent wound infection is to _____.

26. Whenever a wound is irrigated with a solution other than water or normal saline, it is usually _____

_____.

27. When irrigating a wound _____ must be used.

© 1994 W.B. Saunders Company. *Rambo's Nursing Skills for Clinical Practice,* fourth edition
All rights reserved.

28. A penrose drain is a _____.

29. Wound drains generally exit through a _____.

30. Closed drainage systems must be _____ periodically in order to work.

31. When exudate needs to be cultured, the specimen should be taken from _____.

32. When removing sutures from a large incision, it is best to first _____.

33. If dehiscence occurs, the area should be covered with _____.

34. The first step in treating a pressure ulcer is to _____.

35. If the area is a Stage I pressure ulcer, all that may be needed is a _____.

36. A non-infected Stage II pressure ulcer should be cleansed with _____ only.

37. In Stage III and Stage IV pressure ulcers _____ must be debrided before healing can take place.

38. In wound care, promote healing with _____.

39. When moisture is needed in the wound, it is best to use a _____ rather than a wet-to-dry dressing.

40. For Stage III and Stage IV pressure ulcers, the best dressings to use are:

    a. _____

    b. _____

41. Strict _____ is necessary when changing a sterile dressing.

42. When dressing a large abdominal wound where dressings must be changed frequently, it is best to use

    _____ to hold the dressing in place.

© 1994 W.B. Saunders Company. *Rambo's Nursing Skills for Clinical Practice,* fourth edition
All rights reserved.

43. Two factors that will assist the patient with wound healing are:

    a. _____

    b. _____

44. Besides visually assessing a wound, the nurse should also _____ the wound.

45. When considering materials to use in wound dressings, the nurse should ask the patient about allergy to _____.

III. Take the post-test included at the end of the chapter in the text.

© 1994 W.B. Saunders Company. *Rambo's Nursing Skills for Clinical Practice,* fourth edition
All rights reserved.

PERFORMANCE CHECKLIST

Skill 33-1   Sterile dressing change

Student: _____

Date: _____

	Satisfactory	Unsatisfactory
1. Carries out Standard Steps A, B, C, D, and E as indicated.	❑	❑
2. Loosens tape or binder, puts on gloves and removes old dressing.	❑	❑
3. Inspects dressing and places it in discard bag.	❑	❑
4. Removes and discards gloves.	❑	❑
5. Washes hands and puts on sterile gloves.	❑	❑
6. Cleans around the wound with sterile technique.	❑	❑
7. Applies medication if ordered.	❑	❑
8. Applies sterile dressing with sterile technique.	❑	❑
9. Removes gloves and secures dressing.	❑	❑
10. Carries out Standard Steps X, Y, and Z.	❑	❑

Pass _____

Fail _____

Comments: _____

_____

Instructor: _____

© 1994 W.B. Saunders Company. *Rambo's Nursing Skills for Clinical Practice,* fourth edition
All rights reserved.

PERFORMANCE CHECKLIST

Skill 33-2   Wound irrigation

Student: _____

Date: _____

	Satisfactory	Unsatisfactory
1. Carries out Standard Steps A, B, C, D, and E as indicated.	❏	❏
2. Exposes wound using aseptic technique.	❏	❏
3. Prepares irrigation set and places underpad appropriately; places basin to catch irrigation fluid.	❏	❏
4. Washes hands and puts on sterile gloves.	❏	❏
5. Irrigates wound with sterile technique.	❏	❏
6. Dries skin before applying dressing.	❏	❏
7. Applies sterile dressing.	❏	❏
8. Removes and discards gloves.	❏	❏
9. Carries out Standard Steps X, Y, and Z.	❏	❏

Pass _____

Fail _____

Comments: _____

_____

Instructor: _____

© 1994 W.B. Saunders Company. *Rambo's Nursing Skills for Clinical Practice,* fourth edition
All rights reserved.

PERFORMANCE CHECKLIST

Skill 33-3   Care of drainage devices

Student: _____

Date: _____

	Satisfactory	Unsatisfactory
1. Carries out Standard Steps A, B, C, D, and E as indicated.	❑	❑
2. Checks system for proper function; empties with aseptic technique as needed.	❑	❑
3. Measures drainage using universal precautions, records on I & O sheet.	❑	❑
4. Cleanses port, recompresses suction device.	❑	❑
5. Checks drain tubes and connections.	❑	❑
6. Charts characteristics and amount of drainage.	❑	❑
7. Carries out Standard Steps X, Y, and Z.	❑	❑

Pass _____

Fail _____

Comments: _____

_____

Instructor: _____

© 1994 W.B. Saunders Company. *Rambo's Nursing Skills for Clinical Practice,* fourth edition
All rights reserved.

PERFORMANCE CHECKLIST

Skill 33-4   Wet-to-moist or damp dressings

Student: _____

Date: _____

	Satisfactory	Unsatisfactory
1. Carries out Standard Steps A, B, C, D, and E as indicated.	❑	❑
2. Sets up equipment in logical order.	❑	❑
3. Using universal precautions, removes old dressing, inspects it, and discards appropriately.	❑	❑
4. Removes gloves; washes hands and pours wetting solution into sterile basin.	❑	❑
5. Puts on sterile gloves.	❑	❑
6. Wets dressings and wrings them out.	❑	❑
7. Fluffs gauze to be packed in wound.	❑	❑
8. Packs wound and covers with second moist dressing.	❑	❑
9. Places dry dressing over moist dressings.	❑	❑
10. Removes gloves and discards them.	❑	❑
11. Secures dressings with tape or binder.	❑	❑
12. Carries out Standard Steps X, Y, and Z.	❑	❑

Pass _____

Fail _____

Comments: _____

_____

Instructor: _____

© 1994 W.B. Saunders Company. *Rambo's Nursing Skills for Clinical Practice,* fourth edition
All rights reserved.

PERFORMANCE CHECKLIST

Skill 33-5   Removing sutures or staples

Student: _____

Date: _____

	Satisfactory	Unsatisfactory
1. Carries out Standard Steps A, B, C, D, and E as indicated.	❏	❏
2. Removes dressing using universal precautions.	❏	❏
3. Opens suture removal kit.	❏	❏
4. Uses forceps and scissors or staple remover to remove sutures or staples.	❏	❏
5. Cuts sutures opposite knot.	❏	❏
6. Releases staple completely before lifting it free.	❏	❏
7. Removes every other suture or staple first.	❏	❏
8. If wound does not separate, removes other sutures or staples.	❏	❏
9. Cleans site with alcohol swabs.	❏	❏
10. Removes gloves and discards appropriately.	❏	❏
11. Applies steri-strips if ordered.	❏	❏
12. Applies sterile dressing if ordered.	❏	❏
13. Carries out Standard Steps X, Y, and Z.	❏	❏

Pass _____

Fail _____

Comments: _____

_____

Instructor: _____

© 1994 W.B. Saunders Company. *Rambo's Nursing Skills for Clinical Practice,* fourth edition
All rights reserved.

PERFORMANCE CHECKLIST

Skill 33-6 Applying a transparent film dressing

Student: _____

Date: _____

	Satisfactory	Unsatisfactory
1. Carries out Standard Steps A, B, C, D, and E as indicated.	❏	❏
2. Removes old dressing carefully, utilizing universal precautions.	❏	❏
3. Cleanses wound as needed, using sterile technique.	❏	❏
4. Dries and prepares skin around wound.	❏	❏
5. Carefully applies transparent film dressing smoothly.	❏	❏
6. Carries out Standard Steps X, Y, and Z.	❏	❏

Pass _____

Fail _____

Comments: _____

_____

Instructor: _____

© 1994 W.B. Saunders Company. *Rambo's Nursing Skills for Clinical Practice,* fourth edition
All rights reserved.

PERFORMANCE CHECKLIST

Skill 33-7   Application of a hydrocolloid dressing

Student: _____

Date: _____

	Satisfactory	Unsatisfactory
1. Carries out Standard Steps A, B, C, D, and E as indicated.	❏	❏
2. Clip excess hair around wound and cleanse the wound using sterile technique.	❏	❏
3. If wound is deep, uses granules, powder or paste in interior space before applying dressing.	❏	❏
4. Prepares the skin around the border of the wound with skin prep.	❏	❏
5. Applies dressing smoothly and allows a 1" border.	❏	❏
6. Checks dressing for adherence on all borders.	❏	❏
7. Carries out Standard Steps X, Y, and Z.	❏	❏

Pass _____

Fail _____

Comments: _____

_____

Instructor: _____

© 1994 W.B. Saunders Company. *Rambo's Nursing Skills for Clinical Practice,* fourth edition
All rights reserved.

Suggested Clinical Activities

1. Discuss with other nurses on your assigned unit what methods of wound care seem to work the best.

2. Ask to accompany a nurse who is caring for a patient with a pressure ulcer.

3. Read the hospital procedure for care of the various stages of pressure ulcers.

4. Practice sterile dressing changes in the skill lab or in a home simulated situation until you are comfortable and confident of your sterile technique.

5. Seek assignment to patients who need sterile dressing changes.

© 1994 W.B. Saunders Company. *Rambo's Nursing Skills for Clinical Practice,* fourth edition
All rights reserved.

Chapter 34

Preparation for Drug Administration

LEARNING ACTIVITIES

I. Fill in the blank(s) with the correct word(s) or phrase.

1. To prepare for drug administration, the nurse needs to:

   a. _____

   b. _____

   c. _____

   d. _____

2. For the medication treatment to be effective the patient must _____.

3. Drug orders may designate a drug by _____, _____, _____,

   or _____ name.

4. Four possible sources from which a nurse can obtain information about a drug are:

   a. _____

   b. _____

   c. _____

   d. _____

5. The effectiveness of drugs depend on _____.

6. Basically, drugs act by either _____ or _____ cell functions.

7. Factors that affect the rate of drug absorption in an individual include (name at least five)

a. _____

b. _____

c. _____

d. _____

e. _____

8. In most states, drugs can be prescribed by _____, _____, and

_____.

9. In some states _____ can also prescribe some drugs under certain conditions.

10. The role of the nurse is to _____ at a specified time.

11. The current law covering narcotics and drugs subject to abuse is _____

_____.

12. Most "street" drugs come under Schedule _____ of the Controlled Substance Act.

13. Schedule II and III drugs are dispensed to the nursing units and are kept _____

_____.

14. Proof of Use sheets are used _____.

15. Scheduled drugs are counted _____ by _____.

16. Medications should always be given by _____

_____.

17. Medications other than nitroglycerin tablets are not to be _____

_____.

© 1994 W.B. Saunders Company. *Rambo's Nursing Skills for Clinical Practice,* fourth edition
All rights reserved.

18. The five rights of drug administration are:

    a. _____

    b. _____

    c. _____

    d. _____

    e. _____

19. Documentation of drug administration should be done _____.

20. Since the nurse must know about the drug being administered, knowledge about _____ _____ is necessary.

21. Patients are warned not to take dairy products within _____ of taking _____ _____.

22. All medication administration sheets (MARs) should be checked for accuracy at least _____ _____.

23. When teaching patients about their drugs, the nurse covers _____ _____.

24. When a patient questions a dose about to be administered, the nurse should _____ _____.

25. Knowing the action of a drug makes figuring out its _____ much easier.

26. Considering uses of a particular drug, the nurse can often prevent a medication error by asking _____.

27. Side effects are considered _____ when they are detrimental to the patient.

28. The "nursing implications/considerations" section in a drug book tells the nurse _____ _____.

© 1994 W.B. Saunders Company. *Rambo's Nursing Skills for Clinical Practice,* fourth edition
All rights reserved.

29. The reason that the nurse must be familiar with the dosage range for the drug is _____
    _____.

30. When administering a drug to a patient, the nurse should tell _____ and
    _____.

31. Four types of drug preparations that cannot be crushed for a patient who has difficulty swallowing are:

    a. _____

    b. _____

    c. _____

    d. _____

32. When in doubt as to whether a drug should be crushed or not the nurse should _____
    _____.

33. In order to maintain consistent drug levels in the blood, each drug should be administered _____
    _____.

34. To prevent medication errors, each medication should be checked _____.

35. If a patient states "I've never had this pill before," the nurse should _____.

36. Drug dosages often need to be altered for the elderly patient because _____
    _____ and_____ levels may occur.

37. It is very important to have the elderly patient sit upright to take oral medications because
    _____.

38. A particular problem for elderly home care patients is medication containers with _____.

39. It is particularly important to remind the home care patient to always _____ before
    taking any over -the-counter medications or other old prescriptions.

© 1994 W.B. Saunders Company. *Rambo's Nursing Skills for Clinical Practice,* fourth edition
All rights reserved.

40. Most medication errors can be prevented by _____

_____.

II. *Perform the following dosage calculations showing all steps of the calulation.*

1. Give Digoxin 0.125 mg. You have on hand Digoxin 0.25 mg. tablets. You give _____

2. Give liquid Benadryl 35 mg. On hand is a bottle of Benadryl 50 mg/20 cc. You give _____

3. Tylenol gr v is ordered. On hand is Tylenol 150 mg/5ccs. How many teaspoons will you give? _____

4. Give Penicillin G 1 Gm. On hand are Penicillin G 500 mg. tablets. You give _____

5. Add 20 mEq to 1000 mL of D5W. On hand is a vial of KCl with 40 mEq/20 cc. You add _____ ccs to the IV bag.

6. Give Atropine Sulfate 0.4 mg. On hand is a vial of Atropine Sulfate gr. 1/150 per cc. You give _____ cc.

7. Give 1/6 gr. Morphine. On hand is a vial labeled 15 mg/cc. You give _____ cc.

8. Give Heparin Sodium 12,000 U. subq. On hand is Heparin Sodium 10,000 U/cc. You give _____ cc.

9. Give Procaine Penicillin 1,200,000 U I.M. On hand is a vial containing Procain Penicillin labeled 800,000 U/mL. You give _____ cc's.

10. A 22 lb. infant is to receive Ampicillin, 0.5 mg/kg. How many milligrams of Ampicillin do you give? _____

III. *Take the post-test included at the end of the chapter in the text.*

© 1994 W.B. Saunders Company. *Rambo's Nursing Skills for Clinical Practice,* fourth edition
All rights reserved.

PERFORMANCE CHECKLIST

Skill 34-1   Locating information about a drug

Student: _____

Date: _____

	Satisfactory	Unsatisfactory
1. Utilizes a drug reference book.	❑	❑
2. Efficiently looks up drug, gathering information necessary for safe administration.	❑	❑
3. Can identify the signs and symptoms of adverse effects that must be assessed before giving a dose of the drug.	❑	❑
4. Returns the drug reference to its proper location.	❑	❑

Pass _____

Fail _____

Comments: _____

_____

Instructor: _____

© 1994 W.B. Saunders Company. *Rambo's Nursing Skills for Clinical Practice,* fourth edition
All rights reserved.

PERFORMANCE CHECKLIST

Skill 34-2 Calculating dosage for correct administration of a drug

Student: _____

Date: _____

	Satisfactory	Unsatisfactory
1. Utilizes one formula and method consistently for calculating drug dosages.	❑	❑
2. Performs any conversion needed for the problem correctly.	❑	❑
3. Performs the dosage calculation correctly.	❑	❑
4. Determines if the answer is logical.	❑	❑

Pass _____

Fail _____

Comments: _____

_____

Instructor: _____

© 1994 W.B. Saunders Company. *Rambo's Nursing Skills for Clinical Practice*, fourth edition
All rights reserved.

Suggested Clinical Activities

1. Go to a bookstore and compare several Nursing Drug Handbooks; choose the one you find easiest to use.

2. For every assigned clinical patient, make a list of the ordered medications and look them up in the drug handbook, noting nursing implications that are very specific to the particular drug. Consider possible interactions among the drugs on the list for each patient.

3. Practice calculating drug dosages. If you have difficulty in this area, check out a nursing math text from the library and use it. Consult with the instructor.

4. Practice administering medications in the skill lab setting with a peer.

5. Seek opportunities to administer all types of medications when on the clinical unit. If you need injection practice, announce that fact in report and ask that you be called if an injection is needed for any patient on the floor. Remember you must be supervised when giving an injection.

© 1994 W.B. Saunders Company. *Rambo's Nursing Skills for Clinical Practice,* fourth edition
All rights reserved.

Oral, Topical and Inhalant Medications

Chapter 35

LEARNING ACTIVITIES

I. Vocabulary. Insert the appropriate word or abbreviation in the sentence from the vocabulary list.

Vocabulary

EC	OU
instillation	PO
meniscus	subling
OD	supp
OS	topical

1. An order to put drops in the left eye would read " 1 drop _____ after meals and at bedtime.

2. For an oral medication the order reads, 1 tab _____ each a.m.

3. Nitroglycerin tablets are ordered to be taken _____.

4. 1 vaginal _____ each night is placed into the vagina.

5. Ointments are _____ medications.

6. Ointment is placed in both eyes when the order reads "ointment _____ at bedtime."

7. A tablet with the designation _____ after it is never crushed.

8. When pouring a dose of cough medicine, the correct amount is measured at the _____ in the medicine cup.

9. An order for placing eye drops in the right eye would read "1 gtt _____ before meals."

10. When performing an _____, you would gently introduce solution into a body cavity.

II. Match the classification in column I with the action of the drug in column II

Column I	Column II
1. anticoagulants	a. Relieve moderate to severe pain
2. antihypertensives	b. Relieve cough
3. diuretics	c. Relieve nausea; control vomiting
4. cardiotonics	d. Relieve obstruction of air
5. opioids	passages
6. sedative, hypnotics	e. Inhibit clotting of blood
7. antitussives	f. Control high blood pressure
8. bronchodilators	g. Reduce edema; increase urinary
9. antiemetics	output
10. antibiotics	h. Strengthen action of the heart
	i. Kill or inhibit growth
	of microorganisms
	j. Promote sleep; relieve anxiety

III. Fill in the blank(s) with the correct word(s) or phrase.

1. One step in correctly administering medications is to _____ the order correctly.

2. Nurses must _____ medication orders tht are ambiguous, incomplete, or unclear in order to prevent errors.

3. Another nursing function related to drug administration is to _____ the effectiveness of the drugs given.

4. A nursing implication when giving opiods is to observe the patient for signs of _____ by checking for a bowel movement.

5. The systems for measuring medication dosage in the United States are the _____ and

   the _____ system.

6. Whenever calculating drug dosages, the nurse should look at the amount determined to be given to see if it is

   _____.

7. The route by which a drug is given depends on the following three factors:

   a. _____

   b. _____

   c. _____

8. Topical medications are applied only to the _____ or _____.

© 1994 W.B. Saunders Company. *Rambo's Nursing Skills for Clinical Practice,* fourth edition
All rights reserved.

9. The five types of drug orders are:

a. _____

b. _____

c. _____

d. _____

e. _____

10. In most hospitals, narcotics orders have a time limit of _____.

11. Antibiotics must be renewed by order every _____ days.

12. Three benefits of the unit dose system of medication administration are:

a. _____

b. _____

c. _____

13. Suppositories are designed for placement in the _____.

14. Irrigations containing medication are most commonly used in the _____.

15. One of the newest methods of medication delivery to the body is the _____ patch.

16. In the adult, ear drops are often used to _____.

17. Nasal sprays are used for "stuffy" nose caused by a cold or _____ symptoms.

18. Throat lozenges are used to _____ a sore throat.

19. Lung medications are often delivered by _____.

20. Hand-held _____ are commonly used to deliver bronchodilators and _____ _____ to the lungs.

21. Before administering a drug to a patient, the nurse must be aware of any _____ the patient has.

© 1994 W.B. Saunders Company. *Rambo's Nursing Skills for Clinical Practice,* fourth edition
All rights reserved.

22. The nurse should check the various medications the patient is to receive for _____.

23. Another consideration when administering oral drugs is whether the drug can be given _____ _____ or must be given with food.

24. For every drug that is to be administered, the nurse should understand the _____ the patient is receiving it.

25. A very important function of the nurse is to _____ about the medications.

IV. Take the post-test included at the end of the chapter in the text.

© 1994 W.B. Saunders Company. *Rambo's Nursing Skills for Clinical Practice,* fourth edition
All rights reserved.

PERFORMANCE CHECKLIST

Skill 35-1   Using the unit dose system

Student: _____

Date: _____

	Satisfactory	Unsatisfactory
1. Verifies that MAR orders have been compared with physician's orders.	❑	❑
2. Prepares cart with supplies and washes hands.	❑	❑
3. Takes medication cart to patient's room.	❑	❑
4. Verifies patient is ready for medications.	❑	❑
5. Performs first check of medications to be given cross-checking the drug name, dosage, route ordered, date and time to be given.	❑	❑
6. Performs a second complete check of each medication.	❑	❑
7. Can verbalize signs and symptoms of adverse effects and any special precautions for each medication to be given.	❑	❑
8. Pours liquid medications correctly.	❑	❑
9. Identifies the patient by checking the I.D. band, comparing name and hospital number to information imprinted on MAR or card.	❑	❑
10. Performs assessment for side effects and special data required before administering the medications.	❑	❑
11. Checks each medication the third time and tells the patient what the medication is for.	❑	❑
12. Pour water for use of patient to take the medications.	❑	❑
13. Positions patient properly.	❑	❑
14. Opens each medication and gives all medications to the patient; observes patient take the medications.	❑	❑
15. Documents medication doses taken.	❑	❑
16. Repeats the process for the next patient.	❑	❑
17. Returns the unit dose cart to the central area when finished.	❑	❑

Pass _____

Fail _____

Comments: _____

_____

Instructor: _____

© 1994 W.B. Saunders Company. *Rambo's Nursing Skills for Clinical Practice*, fourth edition
All rights reserved.

PERFORMANCE CHECKLIST

Skill 35-2   Eye irrigation

Student: _____

Date: _____

	Satisfactory	Unsatisfactory
1. Carries out Standard Steps A, B, C, D and E as need indicates.	❏	❏
2. Places patient supine with head turned in the direction of the affected eye.	❏	❏
3. Places towel underneath the head and positions light for adequate illumination.	❏	❏
4. Dons gloves and cleanses outside of eye.	❏	❏
5. Pulls upper eyelid up and has patient look down.	❏	❏
6. Irrigates the eye holding syringe about 1/2 to 1 inch above the eye; directs flow from inner to outer part of eye.	❏	❏
7. Repeats irrigation process until desired result is achieved or all prescribed solution has been used.	❏	❏
8. Dries face.	❏	❏
9. Carries out Standard Steps X, Y, and Z.	❏	❏

Pass _____

Fail _____

Comments: _____

_____

Instructor: _____

© 1994 W.B. Saunders Company. *Rambo's Nursing Skills for Clinical Practice,* fourth edition
All rights reserved.

PERFORMANCE CHECKLIST

Skill 35-3   Instillation of eye medications

Student: _____

Date: _____

	Satisfactory	Unsatisfactory
1. Carries out Standard Steps A, B, C, D and E as need indicates. (Checks medication; washes hands thoroughly)	❏	❏
2. Positions patient properly for procedure.	❏	❏
3. Exposes the conjunctival sac and drops correct number of drops of medication, or amount of ointment, into the sac.	❏	❏
4. Occludes lacrimal duct for 1–2 minutes.	❏	❏
5. Cautions patient not to clamp eye tightly shut.	❏	❏
6. For ointment, has patient roll eye around.	❏	❏
7. Cleanses excess medication off of eyelid.	❏	❏
8. Carries out Standard Steps X, Y, and Z.	❏	❏

Pass _____

Fail _____

Comments: _____

_____

Instructor: _____

© 1994 W.B. Saunders Company. *Rambo's Nursing Skills for Clinical Practice,* fourth edition
All rights reserved.

PERFORMANCE CHECKLIST

Skill 35-4   Instillation of nasal medications

Student: _____

Date: _____

	Satisfactory	**Unsatisfactory**
1. Carries out Standard Steps A, B, C, D and E as need indicates. (Checks medication)	❑	❑
2. Positions the patient properly for treatment of desired area.	❑	❑
3. Draws up nose drops.	❑	❑
4. Instills drops correctly.	❑	❑
5. Returns dropper to bottle.	❑	❑
6. Has patient remain in position for 2–5 minutes.	❑	❑
7. Carries out Standard Steps X, Y, and Z.	❑	❑

Pass _____

Fail _____

Comments: _____

_____

Instructor: _____

© 1994 W.B. Saunders Company. *Rambo's Nursing Skills for Clinical Practice,* fourth edition
All rights reserved.

PERFORMANCE CHECKLIST

Skill 35-5 Ear irrigation

Student: _____

Date: _____

	Satisfactory	Unsatisfactory
1. Carries out Standard Steps A, B, C, D and E as need indicates.	❏	❏
2. Positions patient in an upright position.	❏	❏
3. Drapes the shoulder and positions the light for adequate illumination.	❏	❏
4. Prepares syringe and solution and positions basin beneath the ear.	❏	❏
5. Straightens the ear canal.	❏	❏
6. Irrigates the canal using gentle flow of solution.	❏	❏
7. Inspects return fluid; repeats procedure as necessary.	❏	❏
8. Verifies that ear canal is clean.	❏	❏
9. Carries out Standard Steps X, Y, and Z.	❏	❏

Pass _____

Fail _____

Comments: _____

_____

Instructor: _____

© 1994 W.B. Saunders Company. *Rambo's Nursing Skills for Clinical Practice,* fourth edition
All rights reserved.

PERFORMANCE CHECKLIST

Skill 35-6 Instillation of ear medications

Student: _____

Date: _____

	Satisfactory	Unsatisfactory
1. Carries out Standard Steps A, B, C, D and E as need indicates. (Checks medication.)	❏	❏
2. Positions the patient supine with the affected ear uppermost.	❏	❏
3. Draws up medication into the dropper.	❏	❏
4. Straightens the ear canal.	❏	❏
5. Instills the medication.	❏	❏
6. Places cotton in the external meatus.	❏	❏
7. Has patient remain in position for 2–5 minutes.	❏	❏
8. Carries out Standard Steps X, Y, and Z.	❏	❏

Pass _____

Fail _____

Comments: _____

_____

Instructor: _____

© 1994 W.B. Saunders Company. *Rambo's Nursing Skills for Clinical Practice,* fourth edition
All rights reserved.

PERFORMANCE CHECKLIST

Skill 35-7 Assisting a patient to use a metered dose inhaler

Student: _____

Date: _____

	Satisfactory	Unsatisfactory
1. Carries out Standard Steps A, B, C, D and E as need indicates. (Checks medication.)	❑	❑
2. Shakes inhaler well and removes mouth piece cover.	❑	❑
3. Has patient hold inhaler upright and place at mouth opening pointing toward back of throat.	❑	❑
4. Has patient take a deep breath and exhale completely; has patient depress the canister while inhaling deeply; instructs to hold breath for 10 seconds before exhaling.	❑	❑
5. Instructs patient to exhale slowly.	❑	❑
6. Shows patient how to wash the inhaler.	❑	❑
7. Carries out Standard Steps X, Y, and Z.	❑	❑

Pass _____

Fail _____

Comments: _____

_____

Instructor: _____

© 1994 W.B. Saunders Company. *Rambo's Nursing Skills for Clinical Practice,* fourth edition
All rights reserved.

PERFORMANCE CHECKLIST

Skill 35-8   Instillation of vaginal medications

Student: _____

Date: _____

	Satisfactory	Unsatisfactory
1. Carries out Standard Steps A, B, C, D and E as need indicates.	❏	❏
2. Places patient in dorsal recumbent position.	❏	❏
3. Has patient empty the bladder.	❏	❏
FOR VAGINAL DOUCHE		
4. Prepares douche solution, checking the medication properly; clears air from tubing.	❏	❏
5. Administers the douche with slow steady stream, rotating the nozzle periodically.	❏	❏
6. Removes the nozzle and dries the perineum.	❏	❏
FOR VAGINAL SUPPOSITORY		
7. Illuminates the vaginal area.	❏	❏
8. Removes wrapper from suppository and lubricates with water soluble lubricant.	❏	❏
9. Lubricates the index finger, opens labial folds and inserts rounded end of the suppository deep into the vagina.	❏	❏
FOR VAGINAL CREAM OR FOAM		
10. Fills applicator following package insert.	❏	❏
11. Separates labial folds and inserts applicator correct distance into vagina; deposits the medication.	❏	❏
12. Removes the applicator.	❏	❏
13. Cleanses the perineum.	❏	❏
14. Cleanses applicator, if reusable.	❏	❏
15. Has patient remain supine for at least 10 minutes.	❏	❏
16. Places per-pad to catch drainage of medication.	❏	❏
17. Carries out Standard Steps X, Y, and Z.	❏	❏

Pass _____

Fail _____

Comments: _____

_____

Instructor: _____

© 1994 W.B. Saunders Company. *Rambo's Nursing Skills for Clinical Practice,* fourth edition
All rights reserved.

PERFORMANCE CHECKLIST

Skill 35-9 Application of topical medications to the skin

Student: _____

Date: _____

	Satisfactory	Unsatisfactory
1. Carries out Standard Steps A, B, C, D and E as need indicates. (Checks medication.)	❏	❏

TO APPLY LOTION

	Satisfactory	Unsatisfactory
2. Prepare work surface and shake lotion.	❏	❏
3. Moisten gauze or cotton balls using aseptic technique.	❏	❏
4. Apply the liquid to the affected area by patting.	❏	❏
5. Discards gauze or cotton balls correctly, recaps medicine.	❏	❏

FOR APPLICATION OF CREAM OR OINTMENT

	Satisfactory	Unsatisfactory
6. Applies the medication with a gloved finger or a tongue blade correctly.	❏	❏
7. Applies dressing if ordered.	❏	❏

FOR ANTIANGINAL OINTMENT

	Satisfactory	Unsatisfactory
8. Measures correct amount of ointment using paper measuring guide.	❏	❏
9. Applies paper to the patient's skin distributing the ointment beneath the paper gently.	❏	❏
10. Removes all old ointment from previous site.	❏	❏
11. Washes hands after removing gloves.	❏	❏
12. Carries out Standard Steps X, Y, and Z.	❏	❏

Pass _____

Fail _____

Comments: _____

_____

Instructor: _____

© 1994 W.B. Saunders Company. *Rambo's Nursing Skills for Clinical Practice,* fourth edition
All rights reserved.

Suggested Clinical Activities

1. Practice administering oral medications using the unit dose system in the skill lab if available. Use a peer as the "patient".

2. Ask to give medications for at least five patients on a couple of clinical days.

3. Always look up each medication an assigned patient is receiving in order to familiarize yourself with various medications.

4. Seek clinical experiences on various types of nursing units to gain experience in administering all types of medications.

5. Attempt to master information about at least two classifications of drugs per week.

II. Post-test answers are located in the back of the text.

© 1994 W.B. Saunders Company. *Rambo's Nursing Skills for Clinical Practice,* fourth edition
All rights reserved.

Chapter 36

Intradermal, Subcutaneous, and Intramuscular Injections

LEARNING ACTIVITIES

I. Match the item in column I with the type of injection in column II.

Column I

_____ 1. 1 1/2" 20 ga. needle
_____ 2. 1/4" 27 ga. needle
_____ 3. T. B. syringe with 1/4" needle
_____ 4. must form a bleb
_____ 5. placed in tissue above the muscle layer
_____ 6. may be placed in the gluteus medius
_____ 7. 3 ccs of medication
_____ 8. 20 U. of U 100 insulin
_____ 9. 5,000 U. of heparin sodium
_____10. Tuberculin test

Column II

a. intradermal injection
b. subcutaneous
c. intramuscular injection

II. Fill in the blank(s) with the correct word(s) or phrase.

1. Medications given by the parenteral route must be _____,

   and readily _____.

2. Parenteral routes are used for medication administration for the following five reasons:

   a. _____

   b. _____

   c. _____

   d. _____

   e. _____

3. When administering a parenteral injection, the nurse must take the following precautions:

   a. _____

   b. _____

   c. _____

© 1994 W.B. Saunders Company. *Rambo's Nursing Skills for Clinical Practice,* fourth edition   535
All rights reserved.

4. Using the wrong site or route for an injected drug may _____

    _____.

5. To insure proper deposition of the medication in the proper tissue layer, the nurse must select

    _____.

6. When patients are receiving repeated injections, the nurse should _____.

7. When administering an intramuscular injection, it is essential to _____

    before injecting to avoid _____.

8. The intradermal route of injection places small amounts of solution into the _____ layer and is

    mainly used for _____.

9. The subcutaneous injection places the medication _____

    _____.

10. When a 5/8" needle is used for a subcutaneous injection, the angle of injection should be _____.

11. The most frequent sites used for the intramuscular injection are the _____, _____, and

    _____ site and the _____.

12. Up to _____ mL of solution can be injected for an intramuscular injection safely.

13. An _____ drug is absorbed more rapidly than one in an _____.

14. 18 and 19 gauge needles are used for _____ and _____.

15. An intramuscular injection is usually given using a _____, _____, or _____ gauge needle.

16. When withdrawing medication from an ampule, a _____ needle should be used.

17. Universal precautions require that after an injection is given, the syringe and needle be _____

    _____.

© 1994 W.B. Saunders Company. *Rambo's Nursing Skills for Clinical Practice,* fourth edition
All rights reserved.

18. Tuberculin syringes are calibrated to measure _____ of a mL for giving very small doses.

19. Most 3 mL syringes have a scale that measures _____ of a mL.

20. After gathering the equipment and medication, but before beginning to prepare an injection, the nurse should

_____.

21. Parenteral medications come in _____, _____, and _____.

22. Generally, for an IM injection a _____ syringe with a _____ needle is used.

23. Before breaking open an ampule, _____ around the neck.

24. Before opening an ampule, it is necessary to _____.

25. When a drug comes in a powdered form, the solute in the vial is mixed with a _____ before the drug is drawn into a syringe.

26. Typical diluents are _____ and _____.

27. When mixing a powdered drug and then drawing it into a syringe it is necessary to take care to maintain

_____.

28. To prevent coring of a rubber stopper on a vial, the nurse should insert the needle _____

_____.

29. When two drugs are ordered to be given in one injection, the _____ must be checked before drawing them into the syringe.

30. The usual location for giving an intradermal injection is the _____.

© 1994 W.B. Saunders Company. *Rambo's Nursing Skills for Clinical Practice,* fourth edition
All rights reserved.

31. Subcutaneous injections of insulin may be administered into the following sites:

a. _____

b. _____

c. _____

d. _____

e. _____

32. When administering heparin, the site is not _____ after injecting.

33. An intramuscular injection can be safely given in the following sites:

a. _____

b. _____

c. _____

d. _____

34. Two bony landmarks useful in locating a safe location for an intramuscular injection are:

a. _____

b. _____

35. When preparing an intramuscular injection, the three medication checks are done:

a. _____

b. _____

c. _____

36. Z-track injection technique is used when _____.

37. Symptons of anaphylactic shock include:

a. _____

b. _____

c. _____

d. _____

38. Because injected medications are irretreivable, it is especially important to check _____
before giving the injection.

© 1994 W.B. Saunders Company. *Rambo's Nursing Skills for Clinical Practice,* fourth edition
All rights reserved.

39. A contraindication for using a particular injection site is _____ at the site.

40. Giving injections successfully involves:

a. _____

b. _____

c. _____

d. _____

III. Take the post-test included at the end of the chapter in the text.

© 1994 W.B. Saunders Company. *Rambo's Nursing Skills for Clinical Practice,* fourth edition
All rights reserved.

PERFORMANCE CHECKLIST

Skill 36-1   Preparing the syringe for use

Student: _____

Date: _____

	Satisfactory	Unsatisfactory
1. Gathers equipment and washes hands.	❏	❏
2. Selects correct size of syringe and needle; removes outer wrapper.	❏	❏
FOR TUBEX CARTRIDGE		
3. Puts cartridge into holder correctly.	❏	❏
4. Checks medication with MAR using 5 rights.	❏	❏
5. Calculates dosage as necessary.	❏	❏
6. Removes excess medication if necessary.	❏	❏
7. When finished deposits cartridge in sharps container. (disassembles holder & cartridge)	❏	❏

Pass   _____

Fail   _____

Comments: _____

_____

Instructor: _____

© 1994 W.B. Saunders Company. *Rambo's Nursing Skills for Clinical Practice,* fourth edition
All rights reserved.

PERFORMANCE CHECKLIST

Skill 36-2   Withdrawing medication from an ampule

Student: _____

Date: _____

	Satisfactory	Unsatisfactory
1. Gathers equipment and washes hands.	❏	❏
2. Compares medication order with the MAR.	❏	❏
3. Obtains correct medication ampule and performs medication check according to 5 rights.	❏	❏
4. Dislodges the fluid from the stem of the ampul.	❏	❏
5. Breaks the neck of the ampule without cutting skin.	❏	❏
6. Efficiently draws medication dose out of ampule using filtered needle.	❏	❏
7. Expels air from syringe.	❏	❏
8. Leaves exact dosage in syringe.	❏	❏
9. Verifies dosage with MAR; calculates if necessary.	❏	❏
10. Recaps needle when finished drawing up medication.	❏	❏
11. Cleans work area.	❏	❏

Pass _____

Fail _____

Comments: _____

_____

Instructor: _____

© 1994 W.B. Saunders Company. *Rambo's Nursing Skills for Clinical Practice,* fourth edition
All rights reserved.

PERFORMANCE CHECKLIST

Skill 36-3 Withdrawing medication from a vial

Student: _____

Date: _____

		Satisfactory	Unsatisfactory
1.	Gathers equipment and washes hands.	❏	❏
2.	Compares the medication order with the MAR.	❏	❏
3.	Obtains vial of medication and calculates dosage if necessary.	❏	❏
4.	Performs medication check using the five rights.	❏	❏
5.	Opens the vial and swabs the top with alcohol.	❏	❏
6.	Injects air into vial; withdraws medication.	❏	❏
7.	Verifies dose and expels excess air.	❏	❏
8.	Replaces needle guard.	❏	❏
9.	Rechecks medication using the 5 rights.	❏	❏
10.	Cleans up the work area.	❏	❏
11.	Takes the medication to the patient's room.	❏	❏

Pass _____

Fail _____

Comments: _____

_____

Instructor: _____

© 1994 W.B. Saunders Company. *Rambo's Nursing Skills for Clinical Practice,* fourth edition
All rights reserved.

PERFORMANCE CHECKLIST

Skill 36-4 Preparation of medications for injection

Student: _____

Date: _____

	Satisfactory	Unsatisfactory
1. Gathers equipment and washes hands.	❏	❏
2. Checks the MAR with the order sheet.	❏	❏
3. Obtains medication and calculates dosage if necessary.	❏	❏
4. Verifies medication using the 5 rights.	❏	❏
5. Selects proper size needle and syringe.	❏	❏
6. Using aseptic technique, draws up the medication.	❏	❏
7. Verifies exact dosage and recaps needle.	❏	❏
8. Rechecks medication using the 5 rights.	❏	❏

FOR RECONSTITUTION

	Satisfactory	Unsatisfactory
9. Uses proper diluent in correct amount.	❏	❏
10. Mixes drug and solution thoroughly.	❏	❏
11. Changes needle after drawing up the solution.	❏	❏

FOR MIXING 2 DRUGS FROM VIALS OR AMPULES

	Satisfactory	Unsatisfactory
12. Determines drugs are compatible.	❏	❏
13. Calculates total amount to be given and decides on one or two injections.	❏	❏
14. Draws up both medications in the correct order.	❏	❏
15. Obtains exact volume desired for both drugs.	❏	❏

FOR COMBINING DRUGS IN CARTRIDGES

	Satisfactory	Unsatisfactory
16. Determines drugs are compatible.	❏	❏
17. Figures total volume and obtains correct syringe.	❏	❏
18. Adjusts medication in each cartridge to exact dose desired.	❏	❏
19. Places both drugs into one syringe using aseptic technique.	❏	❏
20. Reattaches needle; verifies total volume.	❏	❏
21. Rechecks medications with the MAR using the 5 rights.	❏	❏

© 1994 W.B. Saunders Company. *Rambo's Nursing Skills for Clinical Practice,* fourth edition
All rights reserved.

22. Cleans up work area.   ❑   ❑

23. Takes injection and identifying sheet or card to patient's room, washes hands, dons gloves, identifies patient correctly, and gives injection.   ❑   ❑

24. Disposes of syringe and needle by dropping them into a sharps container.   ❑   ❑

Pass _____

Fail _____

Comments: _____

_____

Instructor: _____

© 1994 W.B. Saunders Company. *Rambo's Nursing Skills for Clinical Practice,* fourth edition
All rights reserved.

PERFORMANCE CHECKLIST

Skill 36-5   Administering an intradermal injection

Student: _____

Date: _____

	Satisfactory	Unsatisfactory
1. Carries out Standard Steps A, B, C, D and E as need indicates.	❑	❑
2. Checks the medication with the MAR using the 5 rights.	❑	❑
3. Draws up the medication correctly.	❑	❑
4. Rechecks the medication using the 5 rights.	❑	❑
5. Properly identifies the patient.	❑	❑
6. Dons gloves and cleanses the injection area.	❑	❑
7. Gives injection and forms bleb.	❑	❑
8. Carries out Standard Steps X, Y, and Z.	❑	❑

Pass   _____

Fail   _____

Comments: _____

_____

Instructor: _____

© 1994 W.B. Saunders Company. *Rambo's Nursing Skills for Clinical Practice,* fourth edition
All rights reserved.

PERFORMANCE CHECKLIST

Skill 36-6   Administering a subcutaneous injection

Student: _____

Date: _____

	Satisfactory	Unsatisfactory
1. Carries out Standard Steps A, B, C, D and E as need indicates.	❏	❏
2. Prepares the medication following the 5 rights.	❏	❏
3. Properly identifies the patient.	❏	❏
4. Dons gloves and selects appropriate site.	❏	❏
5. Cleanses site and administers injection correctly.	❏	❏
6. Removes needle quickly and massages site.	❏	❏
10. Carries out Standard Steps X, Y, and Z.	❏	❏

Pass _____

Fail _____

Comments: _____

_____

Instructor: _____

© 1994 W.B. Saunders Company. *Rambo's Nursing Skills for Clinical Practice,* fourth edition
All rights reserved.

PERFORMANCE CHECKLIST

Skill 36-7   Administering an intramuscular injection

Student: _____

Date: _____

	Satisfactory	**Unsatisfactory**
1. Carries out Standard Steps A, B, C, D and E as need indicates.	❏	❏
2. Verifies the medication with the MAR using the 5 rights.	❏	❏
3. Draws up the medication correctly.	❏	❏
4. Rechecks the medication using the 5 rights.	❏	❏
5. Properly identifies the patient.	❏	❏
6. Chooses appropriate location and utilizes correct landmarks for site.	❏	❏
7. Dons gloves, cleanses area, and gives injection correctly.	❏	❏
8. Removes needle quickly and massages area.	❏	❏
9. Carries out Standard Steps X, Y, and Z.	❏	❏

Pass _____

Fail _____

Comments: _____

_____

Instructor: _____

© 1994 W.B. Saunders Company. *Rambo's Nursing Skills for Clinical Practice,* fourth edition
All rights reserved.

PERFORMANCE CHECKLIST

Skill 36-8   Administering a Z-Track injection

Student: _____

Date: _____

	Satisfactory	Unsatisfactory
1. Carries out Standard Steps A, B, C, D and E as need indicates.	❏	❏
2. Verify the medication with the MAR using the 5 rights.	❏	❏
3. Calculates dosage correctly.	❏	❏
4. Draws up medication correctly using proper equipment.	❏	❏
5. Properly identifies the patient.	❏	❏
6. Dons gloves, selects site using correct landmarks.	❏	❏
7. Pulls skin and tissue laterally.	❏	❏
8. Gives injection correctly.	❏	❏
9. Waits 10 seconds before removing needle.	❏	❏
10. Removes needle smoothly.	❏	❏
11. Carries out Standard Steps X, Y, and Z.	❏	❏

Pass _____

Fail _____

Comments: _____

_____

Instructor: _____

© 1994 W.B. Saunders Company. *Rambo's Nursing Skills for Clinical Practice,* fourth edition
All rights reserved.

Suggested Clinical Activities

1. Practice giving the various types of injections using a mannequin or injection pad in the skill laboratory if possible. If a skill laboratory is not available, practice drawing up and giving injections using an orange or rubber ball at home.

2. Always palpate bony landmarks when giving a parenteral injection into the gluteus medius or ventrogluteal site. Practice locating the right site on several peers or family members of varying weights and sizes.

3. Seek injection experience in the clinical setting by asking in report for the opportunity to give any injections that are needed during the shift.

4. Ask to be assigned to the Day surgery department and/or the Emergency room to obtain injection practice.

© 1994 W.B. Saunders Company. *Rambo's Nursing Skills for Clinical Practice,* fourth edition
All rights reserved.

Chapter 37

Intravenous Medications and Infusions

LEARNING ACTIVITIES

I. Vocabulary. Fill in the appropriate word in the sentence from the vocabulary list.

   Vocabulary

   bolus   infiltrated
   bore   isotonic
   embolus   TPN
   hypertonic   VAD

1. A danger when changing IV solutions on a central line is the risk of air _____.

2. The administration of red blood cells is best done with a large _____ cannula.

3. When a patient experiences the cardiac dysrhythmia ventricular tachycardia, a _____ of lidocaine is given.

4. Normal saline, 0.9% NS, is an _____ solution that neither draws fluid into the vascular compartment, or causes it fluid to disperse out of the vascular compartment.

5. PICC lines, cental lines, implanted ports are all types of _____.

6. _____ is used for nutritional supplementation and the fluids and infusion line must be handled aseptically.

7. Mannitol, sometimes given to reduce intracranial pressure, is a _____ solution.

8. When an intravenous line has _____ the IV site must be changed.

II. Fill in the blank(s) with the correct word(s) or phrase.

1. Intravenous fluids are given to _____ or to _____

_____.

2. Veins in the legs or feet of adults are rarely used for infusion of intravenous solutions because of the danger of

_____.

3. In infants_____ or _____ veins are used for intravenous therapy because veins in the arms and legs are too small.

4. Central line catheters are inserted into the _____ vessel.

5. The average adult needs _____ mL of fluids in a 24 hour period to replace fluids lost by elimination.

6. When drugs are given intravenously, they most often need to be diluted in _____ mL of compatible fluid.

7. Subcutaneous infusion is used for medication for _____.

8. Medication for pain control can also be infused via the _____ or _____ route.

9. An intravenous solution of 5 percent dextrose in water provides _____ calories.

10. Ringer's solution contains normal saline with _____ and _____.

11. TPN solution consists of _____.

12. Solutions given IV may be _____ depending on the needs of the patient and the purpose of the IV.

13. Filters on IV lines have greatly reduced the incidence of _____ by removing bacteria, fungi, and particulates.

14. Filters are also designed to vent _____ from the IV tubing.

15. When selecting an IV bag or bottle, it should be inverted 2–3 times and inspected for _____

_____.

16. When selecting an IV infusion set of tubing, the nurse must check the _____ for the tubing before regulating the IV rate.

17. Microdrop tubing delivers _____ per mL.

© 1994 W.B. Saunders Company. *Rambo's Nursing Skills for Clinical Practice,* fourth edition
All rights reserved.

18. Regular drop tubing delivers _____ per mL.

19. When hanging a piggy-back solution, the container should be hung _____

_____.

20. An advantage of the prn lock or INT lock is that _____

_____.

21. A regular IV line can be converted to a prn lock by _____

_____.

22. A _____ infusion set is used to infuse blood products.

23. After a blood infusion, the line must be _____.

24. Use of a controlled volume set insures that _____

_____.

25. Intravenous infusion pumps deliver _____ at a _____.

26. Many infusion pumps alert the nurse when _____

_____.

27. Two disadvantages of infusion pumps are that they:

    a. _____

    b. _____

28. A patient-controlled-analgesia pump, PCA, is programmed to _____

_____.

29. The most common IV catheter used is the _____ catheter because it causes

    less _____.

© 1994 W.B. Saunders Company. *Rambo's Nursing Skills for Clinical Practice,* fourth edition
All rights reserved.

30. The size of the IV catheter or needles used depends on _____

_____.

31. PICC and MLC are used for short-term peripheral therapy where _____

_____.

32. When the patient has a PICC or MLC line in place, the nurse must remember not to _____

_____.

33. Long term central venous catheters are placed by _____ by the physician.

34. Before infusion through a newly placed central line, verification of placement by _____ must be done.

35. Most infusion ports are placed _____.

36. Before performing venipuncture, it is essential to be able to _____.

37. When performing venipuncture, _____ must be worn and _____ must be maintained.

38. It is not good practice to _____ an IV that is running behind schedule.

39. To calculate the rate of flow, the nurse must know the _____ per mL that pass through the drip chamber.

40. Fluids infused faster than _____ mL per hour may cause _____ and lead

to _____.

41. A primary principle of IV therapy is to _____ of the fluid.

42. Another principle is to protect the needle site from _____ which might cause

_____.

43. An IV solution container should not be allowed to _____ before changing to the next one.

© 1994 W.B. Saunders Company. *Rambo's Nursing Skills for Clinical Practice,* fourth edition
All rights reserved.

44. It is essential to remove _____ from the tubing before starting an IV infusion.

45. Whenever a patient is placed on intravenous therapy, _____ recording is also done.

46. Signs of IV infiltration include _____

_____.

47. Reactions to transfusions of blood usually occur _____.

48. The most common signs of transfusion reaction are _____, _____, _____, _____ and _____.

49. A new container of IV solution is usually begun when there is _____ left in the one hanging.

50. Administration of any blood product requires a _____.

III. Calculate the correct flow rate for the following IV orders.

1. 1000 cc D5RL at 125 cc/hour. Drop factor: 15 gtts/cc

2. 250 cc D5W with 20 mEq potassium chloride over 3 hours. Drop factor: 60 gtts/cc

3. 1000 cc NS q 10 hours. Drop factor: 15 gtts/cc

4. 1000 cc D5W 1/2NS q 8 hours. Drop factor: 10 gtts/cc

5. 500 cc D5W at 80 cc/hr. Drop factor: 10 gtts/cc

IV. Take the post-test included at the end of the chapter in the text.

© 1994 W.B. Saunders Company. *Rambo's Nursing Skills for Clinical Practice,* fourth edition
All rights reserved.

PERFORMANCE CHECKLIST

Skill 37-1   Starting the primary IV solution

Student: _____

Date: _____

	Satisfactory	Unsatisfactory
1. Carries out Standard Steps A, B, C, D, and E as need indicates.	❑	❑
2. Checks the IV solution with the order.	❑	❑
3. Checks solution for sterility and expiration date.	❑	❑
4. Attaches IV administration set efficiently without contaminating it.	❑	❑
5. Clears tubing of air without wasting solution.	❑	❑
6. Places time tape label on container and marks it correctly.	❑	❑
7. Re-verifies IV solution and additives, if any, with MAR.	❑	❑
8. Verifies patient identity correctly.	❑	❑
9. Chooses appropriate IV site for infusion.	❑	❑
10. Prepares the IV site properly.	❑	❑
11. Dons gloves and inserts IV cannula or needle.	❑	❑
12. Removes tourniquet and attaches IV tubing; begins infusion.	❑	❑
13. Observes for any problems with infusion.	❑	❑
14. Applies a sterile dressing to IV site; secures tubing to the patient.	❑	❑
15. Protects site with an armboard if needed.	❑	❑
15. Regulates IV flow as ordered.	❑	❑
16. Carries out Standard Steps X, Y, and Z.	❑	❑

Pass _____

Fail _____

Comments: _____

_____

Instructor: _____

© 1994 W.B. Saunders Company. *Rambo's Nursing Skills for Clinical Practice,* fourth edition
All rights reserved.

PERFORMANCE CHECKLIST

Skill 37-2   Adding a new solution to the IV infusion

Student: _____

Date: _____

	Satisfactory	Unsatisfactory
1. Carries out Standard Steps A, B, C, D, and E as need indicates.	❏	❏
2. Checks the solution for sterility and expiration date.	❏	❏
3. Compares label with order.	❏	❏
4. Places a time tape on the solution.	❏	❏
5. Properly identifies patient before adding solution.	❏	❏
6. Removes IV tubing from completed bag and spikes new bag of IV solution.	❏	❏
7. Removes air bubbles that occurred in tubing.	❏	❏
8. Readjusts flow rate to prescribed rate.	❏	❏
9. Disposes of empty container.	❏	❏
10. Records the added fluid on the parenteral infusion record.	❏	❏
11. Carries out Standard Steps X, Y, and Z.	❏	❏

Pass _____

Fail _____

Comments: _____

_____

Instructor: _____

© 1994 W.B. Saunders Company. *Rambo's Nursing Skills for Clinical Practice,* fourth edition
All rights reserved.

PERFORMANCE CHECKLIST

Skill 37-3   Adding medication to an IV solution

Student: _____

Date: _____

	Satisfactory	Unsatisfactory
1. Carries out Standard Steps A, B, C, D, and E as need indicates.	❑	❑
2. Checks the medication and the IV solution with the physician's order.	❑	❑
3. Prepares additive label for medication.	❑	❑
4. Prepares the medication and draws it up into a syringe.	❑	❑
5. Removes tab from medication injection port and injects medication into the IV solution.	❑	❑
6. Places additive label on bag.	❑	❑
7. Mixes the medication and the solution.	❑	❑
8. Re-checks the medication with the MAR order.	❑	❑
9. Carries out Standard Steps X, Y, and Z.	❑	❑

Pass _____

Fail _____

Comments: _____

_____

Instructor: _____

© 1994 W.B. Saunders Company. *Rambo's Nursing Skills for Clinical Practice,* fourth edition
All rights reserved.

PERFORMANCE CHECKLIST

Skill 37-4 IV piggy-back medication (IVPB)

Student: _____

Date: _____

	Satisfactory	Unsatisfactory
1. Carries out Standard Steps A, B, C, D, and E as need indicates.	❏	❏
2. Check the medication with the order; calculate dosage if needed; prepare label.	❏	❏
3. Prepare the medication and draw it up into a syringe.	❏	❏
4. Checks compatibility of medication, IVPB solution with primary IV solution.	❏	❏
5. Injects the medication into the IVPB solution bag.	❏	❏
6. Applies the label and mixes the medication and solution.	❏	❏
7. Hooks up the IVPB administration set to the IVBP bag.	❏	❏
8. Clears air from the tubing without wasting medication.	❏	❏
9. Re-verifies the medication and dosage with the MAR.	❏	❏
10. Properly identifies the patient and verifies any allergies.	❏	❏
11. Attaches the tubing to the cleansed port on the primary infusion set.	❏	❏
12. Adjusts the drop rate of the IVPB to the correct flow.	❏	❏
13. Monitors the patient closely	❏	❏
14. Carries out Standard Steps X, Y, and Z.	❏	❏

Pass _____

Fail _____

Comments: _____

_____

Instructor: _____

© 1994 W.B. Saunders Company. *Rambo's Nursing Skills for Clinical Practice,* fourth edition
All rights reserved.

PERFORMANCE CHECKLIST

Skill 37-5   Medication administration via a volume-control set (burette)

Student: _____

Date: _____

	Satisfactory	Unsatisfactory
1. Carries out Standard Steps A, B, C, D, and E as need indicates.	❏	❏
2. Checks the medication with the MAR order.	❏	❏
3. Prepares the medication and draws it up in a syringe.	❏	❏
4. Properly identifies the patient; re-verifies the medication with the MAR.	❏	❏
5. Cleanses the injection cap on the burette and adds the medication to the correct amount of IV solution.	❏	❏
6. Labels the burette and mixes the medication and solution.	❏	❏
7. Opens lower clamp and adjusts the rate of flow.	❏	❏
8. As soon as burette empties, reopens top clamp to continue the IV infusion.	❏	❏
9. Carries out Standard Steps X, Y, and Z.	❏	❏

Pass   _____

Fail   _____

Comments: _____

_____

Instructor: _____

© 1994 W.B. Saunders Company. *Rambo's Nursing Skills for Clinical Practice,* fourth edition
All rights reserved.

PERFORMANCE CHECKLIST

Skill 37-6   Intravenous bolus medication administration

Student: _____

Date: _____

	Satisfactory	**Unsatisfactory**
1. Carries out Standard Steps A, B, C, D, and E as need indicates.	❏	❏
2. Checks the medication with the physician's order.	❏	❏
3. Prepares the medication; checks compatibility with the IV solution infusing.	❏	❏
4. Properly identifies the patient.	❏	❏
5. Cleanses the injection port and administers the medication over correct time period.	❏	❏
6. Observes for adverse reactions.	❏	❏
7. Allows primary IV infusion to continue, or flushes "prn" lock.	❏	❏
8. Carries out Standard Steps X, Y, and Z.	❏	❏

Pass _____

Fail _____

Comments: _____

_____

Instructor: _____

© 1994 W.B. Saunders Company. *Rambo's Nursing Skills for Clinical Practice,* fourth edition
All rights reserved.

PERFORMANCE CHECKLIST

Skill 37-7   Intermittent IV or "prn" lock

Student: _____

Date: _____

	Satisfactory	**Unsatisfactory**
1. Carries out Standard Steps A, B, C, D, and E as need indicates.	❏	❏
2. Selects an appropriate site for insertion.	❏	❏
3. Inserts IV cannula or needle.	❏	❏
4. Injects 2 ml of normal saline.	❏	❏
5. Secures the lock with a dressing.	❏	❏
6. Prepares the IV medication correctly, checking the medication with the order.	❏	❏
7. Cleanses the injection cap each time before inserting the needle.	❏	❏
8. Re-verifies the medication again with the MAR.	❏	❏
9. Properly identifies patient.	❏	❏
10. Injects medication over correct time period;	❏	❏
11. Flushes the lock according to agency protocol.	❏	❏
12. Carries out Standard Steps X, Y, and Z.	❏	❏

Pass   _____

Fail   _____

Comments: _____

_____

Instructor: _____

© 1994 W.B. Saunders Company. *Rambo's Nursing Skills for Clinical Practice,* fourth edition
All rights reserved.

PERFORMANCE CHECKLIST

Skill 37-8   Converting an IV needle or cannula to a "prn" lock

Student: _____

Date: _____

	Satisfactory	Unsatisfactory
1. Carries out Standard Steps A, B, C, D, and E as need indicates.	❑	❑
2. Check the physician's order; verify how long the needle or cannula has been at this site.	❑	❑
3. Places a protective pad under the site.	❑	❑
4. Don gloves; prepare the injection cap to place on the cannula.	❑	❑
5. Clamp off the IV infusion, remove the tubing from the cannula and attach the injection cap.	❑	❑
6. Cleanse the area if blood leaked out of the vein.	❑	❑
7. Flush the cannula according to agency policy.	❑	❑
8. Re-dress the IV site.	❑	❑
9. Carries out Standard Steps X, Y, and Z.	❑	❑

Pass _____

Fail _____

Comments: _____

_____

Instructor: _____

© 1994 W.B. Saunders Company. *Rambo's Nursing Skills for Clinical Practice,* fourth edition
All rights reserved.

PERFORMANCE CHECKLIST

Skill 37-9   Discontinuing an IV infusion

Student: _____

Date: _____

	Satisfactory	**Unsatisfactory**
1. Carries out Standard Steps A, B, C, D, and E as need indicates.	❏	❏
2. Verify the order to discontinue the IV.	❏	❏
3. Properly identify the patient and remove the IV dressing.	❏	❏
4. Don gloves; clamp the tubing, and quickly withdraw the IV cannula.	❏	❏
5. Apply pressure to stop the bleeding.	❏	❏
6. Cleanse the area and apply an adhesive bandage.	❏	❏
7. Carries out Standard Steps X, Y, and Z.	❏	❏

Pass _____

Fail _____

Comments: _____

_____

Instructor: _____

© 1994 W.B. Saunders Company. *Rambo's Nursing Skills for Clinical Practice,* fourth edition
All rights reserved.

PERFORMANCE CHECKLIST

Skill 37-10 Obtaining specimens of blood using the Vacutainer system

Student: _____

Date: _____

	Satisfactory	Unsatisfactory
1. Carries out Standard Steps A, B, C, D, and E as need indicates.	❑	❑
2. Prepare the Vacutainer system or syringe and needle.	❑	❑
3. Select a vein.	❑	❑
4. Cleanse the site, don gloves, apply the tourniquet and perform the venipuncture.	❑	❑
5. Draw the blood samples as needed.	❑	❑
6. Is careful not to disrupt the needle when changing collection tubes.	❑	❑
7. Removes needle and applies pressure to puncture site.	❑	❑
8. Labels tubes correctly.	❑	❑
9. Fills out requisition slips and sends specimens to the laboratory.	❑	❑
10. Carries out Standard Steps X, Y, and Z.	❑	❑

Pass _____

Fail _____

Comments: _____

_____

Instructor: _____

© 1994 W.B. Saunders Company. *Rambo's Nursing Skills for Clinical Practice,* fourth edition
All rights reserved.

PERFORMANCE CHECKLIST

Skill 37-11 Infusion of blood products

Student: _____

Date: _____

	Satisfactory	Unsatisfactory
1. Carries out Standard Steps A, B, C, D, and E as need indicates.	❑	❑
2. Verifies size of IV catheter in place.	❑	❑
3. Obtains blood using proper procedure.	❑	❑
4. Double checks the blood with another nurse,	❑	❑
5. Attaches the "Y" administration set and sets up normal saline solution.	❑	❑
6. Spikes the blood component bag correctly.	❑	❑
7. Properly identifies the patient and checks the blood identification bracelet with the transfusion record numbers.	❑	❑
8. Dons gloves and connects the blood component to the administration set.	❑	❑
9. Obtains baseline vital signs.	❑	❑
10. Primes administration set with normal saline.	❑	❑
11. Begins the blood administration, remains with patient for first 5 minutes and checks the patient every 15 minutes for first half hour.	❑	❑
12. Monitors vital signs every 30 minutes.	❑	❑
13. Flushes line with normal saline at end of infusion.	❑	❑
14. Carries out Standard Steps X, Y, and Z.	❑	❑

Pass _____

Fail _____

Comments: _____

_____

Instructor: _____

© 1994 W.B. Saunders Company. *Rambo's Nursing Skills for Clinical Practice,* fourth edition
All rights reserved.

PERFORMANCE CHECKLIST

Skill 37-12   Assisting with the insertion of a central venous catheter

Student: _____

Date: _____

	Satisfactory	Unsatisfactory
1. Carries out Standard Steps A, B, C, D, and E as need indicates.	❑	❑
2. Positions patient correctly.	❑	❑
3. Sets up equipment, maintaining asepsis.	❑	❑
4. Assists the physician with the procedure.	❑	❑
5. Attaches IV tubing and manometer, if used, to the central venous line when it is in place.	❑	❑
6. Adjusts the IV flow rate.	❑	❑
7. Dresses the site correctly.	❑	❑
8. Carries out Standard Steps X, Y, and Z.	❑	❑

Pass _____

Fail _____

Comments: _____

_____

Instructor: _____

© 1994 W.B. Saunders Company. *Rambo's Nursing Skills for Clinical Practice,* fourth edition
All rights reserved.

PERFORMANCE CHECKLIST

Skill 37-13   Measuring central venous pressure

Student: _____

Date: _____

	Satisfactory	**Unsatisfactory**
1. Carries out Standard Steps A, B, C, D, and E as need indicates.	❏	❏
2. Places the patient supine and "zeros" the manometer at the level of the right atrium.	❏	❏
3. Fills the manometer to correct level.	❏	❏
4. Takes CVP reading.	❏	❏
5. Repositions stopcock so that IV fluid infuses into patient.	❏	❏
6. Carries out Standard Steps X, Y, and Z.	❏	❏

Pass _____

Fail _____

Comments: _____

_____

Instructor: _____

© 1994 W.B. Saunders Company. *Rambo's Nursing Skills for Clinical Practice,* fourth edition
All rights reserved.

PERFORMANCE CHECKLIST

Skill 37-14   Changing a central venous catheter dressing and injection cap

Student: _____

Date: _____

	Satisfactory	Unsatisfactory
1. Carries out Standard Steps A, B, C, D, and E as need indicates.	❏	❏
2. Prepares equipment.	❏	❏
3. Uses masks as agency protocol directs.	❏	❏
4. Dons gloves and removes old dressing.	❏	❏
5. Inspects the site for problems.	❏	❏
6. Dons sterile gloves and cleanses site per agency protocol.	❏	❏
7. Applies a new sterile, air-occlusive, dressing.	❏	❏
8. Change the IV tubing and re-tape the catheter and tubing connection.	❏	❏
9. Cleanses connection of injection cap.	❏	❏
10. Dons gloves and clamps catheter	❏	❏
11. Removes old cap and applies new injection cap.	❏	❏
12. Labels the dressing and tubing.	❏	❏
13. Carries out Standard Steps X, Y, and Z.	❏	❏

Pass _____

Fail _____

Comments: _____

_____

Instructor: _____

© 1994 W.B. Saunders Company. *Rambo's Nursing Skills for Clinical Practice,* fourth edition
All rights reserved.

PERFORMANCE CHECKLIST

Skill 37-15   Flushing an implanted infusion port

Student: _____

Date: _____

	Satisfactory	**Unsatisfactory**
1. Carries out Standard Steps A, B, C, D, and E as need indicates.	❑	❑
2. Prepares equipment; labels syringe containing heparin solution.	❑	❑
3. Locates septum of implanted port and cleanses skin for 3-4 inch diameter.	❑	❑
4. Inserts Huber needle firmly into the center of the port.	❑	❑
5. Verifies placement of needle.	❑	❑
6. Flushes and heparinizes the port correctly.	❑	❑
7. Carries out Standard Steps X, Y, and Z.	❑	❑

Pass _____

Fail _____

Comments: _____

_____

Instructor: _____

© 1994 W.B. Saunders Company. *Rambo's Nursing Skills for Clinical Practice,* fourth edition
All rights reserved.

Suggested Clinical Activities

1. Practice changing IV fluid containers in the skill lab with a peer observing your technique. Ask to practice as much as needed until you are comfortable.

2. Practice adding medications to an IV fluid container and calculating the flow rate in the skill lab. Have someone observe your technique and check your calculations.

3. For each assigned clinical patient who has an IV, calculate the flow rate from the order sheet.

4. Practice adjusting the flow rate with the roller clamp in the skill lab setting. Practice until you are comfortable adjusting the rate.

5. Have a staff nurse or your instructor show you how to set up an IV infusion pump.

6. Go with a staff nurse whenever she goes to "trouble-shoot" an infusion pump.

7. Seek opportunities to change IV solutions in the clinical setting by telling the nurses on the unit that you desire this experience and to call you whenever a solution is to be changed. Remember to check the order yourself and to stick to the five rights.

8. Observe other nurses starting IV lines in the clincial setting. Practice IV starts in the skill lab using an IV arm, or seek this practice through the clinical facility education department.

© 1994 W.B. Saunders Company. *Rambo's Nursing Skills for Clinical Practice,* fourth edition
All rights reserved.

Chapter 38

Respiratory Care Techniques

LEARNING ACTIVITIES

I. Vocabulary. Fill in the sentence with the appropriate word from the vocabulary list.

Vocabulary

anoxia	stridor
atelectasis	tachypnea
cyanosis	tenacious
dyspnea	tracheostomy
hypoxia	ventilation

1. The patient with emphysema often experiences _____ with normal daily activities.

2. All patients who have general anesthesia and are on the operating table for a few hours have areas of _____ in the lungs.

3. The patient suffering from hypoxemia may display signs of _____.

4. People who have asthma demonstrate the sounds of _____ during an acute attack.

5. People trapped in burning buildings often suffer _____.

6. The patient in respiratory failure needs mechanical _____.

7. Bronchitis may cause _____ secretions.

8. Patients with pneumonia experience varying degrees of _____.

9. If an upper airway obstruction occurs, the patient may benefit from a _____.

10. The patient who is hypoxic, compensates with _____.

II. Fill in the blank(s) with the correct word(s) or phrase.

1. A top nursing priority for the patient in any situation is _____

    _____ .

2. Although visible signs of dyspnea may indicate hypoxia, more subtle signs are obtained from

    _____   _____ .

3. Oxygen is needed by all cells of the body in order to _____

    _____ .

4. Without oxygen, some cells begin to die in _____ .

5. The most common cause of respiratory insufficiency is _____ .

6. Respiratory insufficiency is defined as _____

    _____ .

7. Five common causes of respiratory insufficiency include:

    a. _____

    b. _____

    c. _____

    d. _____

    e. _____

8. The earliest signs of hypoxemia include _____ .

9. When the oxygen level to the heart muscle is decreased, _____ .

10. Late signs of respiratory failure include _____ .

11. Hypoxia is treated by _____ .

12. Normal body pH is _____ .

© 1994 W.B. Saunders Company. *Rambo's Nursing Skills for Clinical Practice,* fourth edition
All rights reserved.

13. When the body becomes acidotic, the pH _____.

14. The best indicator of adequate gas exchange on the alveolar level is _____.

15. The pulse oximeter measures oxygen saturation by _____

_____.

16. Hypoxia can occur in any person with:

    a. _____

    b. _____

    c. _____

17. In persons with chronic lung disease and carbon dioxide retention, oxygen should be administered in low doses

    because _____

    _____.

18. Patients with respiratory impairment are prone to develop _____.

19. Four basic principles of nursing care for the patient with a respiratory problem include:

    a. _____

    b. _____

    c. _____

    d. _____

20. Postural drainage is used to _____ secretions and promote adequate _____

    _____.

21. It is essential to _____ the patient pre- and post-suctioning.

22. If secretions are difficult copious, the nurse should let the patient _____ between suctioning efforts.

23. When performing endotracheal suctioning, _____ must be maintained.

24. To clear the tubing after endotracheal suctioning, _____ must be used.

© 1994 W.B. Saunders Company. *Rambo's Nursing Skills for Clinical Practice,* fourth edition
All rights reserved.

25. Patients at risk of developing cardiac arrhythmias during suctioning include:

    a. _____

    b. _____

    c. _____

26. Artificial airways may be used to:

    a. _____

    b. _____

    c. _____

    d. _____

27. If an artificial airway is needed for more than a week or ten days, the physician should perform a

    _____.

28. When administering oxygen to a patient, it is the nurse's responsibility to check _____
    of the oxygen.

29. When a patient is on oxygen therapy, oral care should be given _____.

30. When discontinuing oxygen, allow _____ before increasing the patient's activity.

31. When oxygen is in use all electrical equipment must be _____.

32. When oxygen is ordered, it is best for it to be _____ before reaching the patient.

33. The Venturi mask provides oxygen _____.

34. IPPB treatments, when ordered, are given for _____ times a day.

35. Most patients undergoing a tracheostomy are apprehensive and fearful of _____

    _____.

36. It is extremely important the the tracheostomy patient be provided with a means to _____.

© 1994 W.B. Saunders Company. *Rambo's Nursing Skills for Clinical Practice,* fourth edition
All rights reserved.

37. Complications to be assessed for following a tracheostomy include:

    a. _____

    b. _____

    c. _____

38. The patient with a tracheostomy requires a _____, _____ environment.

39. There should always be functioning suction and _____ at the bedside of the patient with a tracheostomy.

40. It is of prime importance that the nurse do everything possible to prevent _____ in the tracheostomy patient.

41. The patient with a tracheostomy is more prone to lung infection because _____

    _____.

42. Before beginning tracheostomy suctioning, the nurse should observe the patient's _____

    _____.

43. Suctioning the tracheostomy should last _____ seconds and no longer than _____.

44. The advantage of an in-line suction catheter is _____.

45. When an inflatable cuff tracheostomy tube is inserted, the pressure in the cuff should be checked every

    _____.

46. Negative pressure ventilators are effective for patients with _____.

47. When the patient is on the ventilator, at the beginning of the shift the nurse must check _____

    _____.

48. The purpose of PEEP is to _____.

49. CPAP is used for patients who _____.

50. The pressure support ventilators assist the patient by _____.

© 1994 W.B. Saunders Company. *Rambo's Nursing Skills for Clinical Practice,* fourth edition
All rights reserved.

51. The chest tube either _____ or _____.

52. Hyperbaric oxygen chambers are currently being used to speed _____.

53. When assessing respirations, the nurse must assess the _____
_____.

54. Slight hypoxia may be reversed by _____.

55. Mucous often is thicker in the elderly patient because _____
_____.

III. Take the post-test included at the end of the chapter in the text.

© 1994 W.B. Saunders Company. *Rambo's Nursing Skills for Clinical Practice,* fourth edition
All rights reserved.

PERFORMANCE CHECKLIST

Skill 38-1 Forced exhalation cough

Student: _____

Date: _____

	Satisfactory	**Unsatisfactory**
1. Carries out Standard Steps A, B, C, D, and E as indicated.	❑	❑
2. Places patient in sitting position with pillow on lap; provides tissues.	❑	❑
3. Has patient deep breathe.	❑	❑
4. Instructs patient to take a deep breath and bend forward while producing a series of coughs upon exhalation.	❑	❑
5. Repeats procedure until cough is nonproductive.	❑	❑
6. Auscultates lungs.	❑	❑
7. Carries out Standard Steps X, Y, and Z.	❑	❑

Pass _____

Fail _____

Comments: _____

_____

Instructor: _____

© 1994 W.B. Saunders Company. *Rambo's Nursing Skills for Clinical Practice,* fourth edition
All rights reserved.

PERFORMANCE CHECKLIST

Skill 38-2   Administering oxygen therapy

Student: _____

Date: _____

	Satisfactory	Unsatisfactory
1. Carries out Standard Steps A, B, C, D, and E as indicated.	❏	❏
2. Connects flowmeter and attaches tubing.	❏	❏
3. Positions oxygen therapy device ordered properly on patient.	❏	❏
4. Adjusts oxygen flow to rate ordered.	❏	❏
5. Carries out Standard Steps X, Y, and Z.	❏	❏

Pass _____

Fail _____

Comments: _____

_____

Instructor: _____

© 1994 W.B. Saunders Company. *Rambo's Nursing Skills for Clinical Practice,* fourth edition
All rights reserved.

PERFORMANCE CHECKLIST

Skill 38-3   Preparation of oxygen cylinder and portable oxygen system

Student: _____

Date: _____

	Satisfactory	Unsatisfactory
1. Carries out Standard Steps A, B, C, D, and E as indicated.	❑	❑
2. Cracks the valve on the oxygen cylinder.	❑	❑
3. Attaches the regulator to the valve outlet.	❑	❑
4. Attaches the tubing.	❑	❑
5. Adjusts the oxygen flow to ordered rate.	❑	❑

Pass _____

Fail _____

Comments: _____

_____

Instructor: _____

© 1994 W.B. Saunders Company. *Rambo's Nursing Skills for Clinical Practice,* fourth edition
All rights reserved.

PERFORMANCE CHECKLIST

Skill 38-4   Nasopharyngeal suctioning

Student: _____

Date: _____

	Satisfactory	Unsatisfactory
1. Carries out Standard Steps A, B, C, D, and E as indicated.	❏	❏
2. Connect tubing to suction source; sets suction pressure correctly.	❏	❏
3. Opens and prepares equipment and supplies.	❏	❏
4. Dons sterile gloves.	❏	❏
5. Attaches catheter to connecting tubing maintaining sterile technique.	❏	❏
6. Moistens catheter and introduces via the nare.	❏	❏
7. Suctions patient for no more than 10 seconds using aseptic technique.	❏	❏
9. Rinses suction catheter.	❏	❏
10. Suctions other nare.	❏	❏
11. Rinses catheter.	❏	❏
12. Asks patient to cough.	❏	❏
13. Suctions oropharynx and mouth	❏	❏
14. Rinses catheter and suction tubing.	❏	❏
15. Disposes of catheter or cleanses and stores catheter aseptically.	❏	❏
16. Carries out Standard Steps X, Y, and Z.	❏	❏

Pass _____

Fail _____

Comments: _____

_____

Instructor: _____

© 1994 W.B. Saunders Company. *Rambo's Nursing Skills for Clinical Practice,* fourth edition
All rights reserved.

PERFORMANCE CHECKLIST

Skill 38-5   Tracheobronchial suctioning

Student: _____

Date: _____

	Satisfactory	Unsatisfactory
1. Carries out Standard Steps A, B, C, D, and E as indicated.	❑	❑
2. Attaches connecting tubing, turns on suction and checks pressure.	❑	❑
3. Opens supplies and dons sterile gloves.	❑	❑
5. Pours solution.	❑	❑
6. Connects catheter to tubing with sterile technique.	❑	❑
7. Pre-oxygenates patient.	❑	❑
8. Moistens catheter.	❑	❑
9. Suctions patient via endotracheal or tracheostomy tube using sterile technique.	❑	❑
10. Suctions for no more than 10 seconds.	❑	❑
11. Reattaches patient to oxygen source.	❑	❑
12. Allows rest period between suctioning.	❑	❑
13. Rinses catheter and tubing.	❑	❑
14. Disposes of catheter and gloves properly.	❑	❑
15. Auscultates lungs to verify success of suctioning.	❑	❑
16. Carries out Standard Steps X, Y, and Z.	❑	❑

Pass _____

Fail _____

Comments: _____

_____

Instructor: _____

© 1994 W.B. Saunders Company. *Rambo's Nursing Skills for Clinical Practice,* fourth edition
All rights reserved.

PERFORMANCE CHECKLIST

Skill 38-6   Tracheostomy care

Student: _____

Date: _____

	Satisfactory	Unsatisfactory
1. Carries out Standard Steps A, B, C, D, and E as indicated.	❑	❑
2. Opens supplies and pours solutions.	❑	❑
3. Using gloves, unlocks the inner cannula and removes it; places it in cleansing solution.	❑	❑
4. Cleans the inner cannula maintaining aseptic technique.	❑	❑
5. Dries the cannula, reinserts it and locks it in place.	❑	❑
6. Removes old dressing and cleans tracheostomy.	❑	❑
7. Replaces tube ties or holder, if soiled, following safety precautions.	❑	❑
8. Applies new pre-cut dressing.	❑	❑
9. Carries out Standard Steps X, Y, and Z.	❑	❑

Pass _____

Fail _____

Comments: _____

_____

Instructor: _____

© 1994 W.B. Saunders Company. *Rambo's Nursing Skills for Clinical Practice,* fourth edition
All rights reserved.

PERFORMANCE CHECKLIST

Skill 38-7   Operation of a mechanical ventilator

Student: _____

Date: _____

	Satisfactory	Unsatisfactory
1. Carries out Standard Steps A, B, C, D, and E as indicated.	❑	❑
2. Checks settings and verifies that they are as ordered: tidal volume, percentage of oxygen, breaths per minute, pressure limits, mode.	❑	❑
3. Checks humidifier and tubing connections.	❑	❑
4. Sets alarms.	❑	❑
5. Checks patient and auscultates lungs to see that proper ventilation is occurring.	❑	❑

Pass _____

Fail _____

Comments: _____

_____

Instructor: _____

© 1994 W.B. Saunders Company. *Rambo's Nursing Skills for Clinical Practice,* fourth edition
All rights reserved.

PERFORMANCE CHECKLIST

Skill 38-8   Monitoring oxygen saturation with a pulse oximeter

Student: _____

Date: _____

	Satisfactory	Unsatisfactory
1. Carries out Standard Steps A, B, C, D, and E as indicated.	❏	❏
2. Sets up and checks oximeter.	❏	❏
3. Applies probe properly and checks for proper reading.	❏	❏
4. Sets alarm.	❏	❏
5. Records data at start and each hour.	❏	❏
6. Turns, coughs and deep breathes patient every 2 hours.	❏	❏
7. Rotates probe, if needed, every 4 hours.	❏	❏
8. Carries out Standard Steps X, Y, and Z.	❏	❏

Pass _____

Fail _____

Comments: _____

_____

Instructor: _____

© 1994 W.B. Saunders Company. *Rambo's Nursing Skills for Clinical Practice,* fourth edition
All rights reserved.

PERFORMANCE CHECKLIST

Skill 38-9   Setting up and monitoring chest tubes and drainage systems

Student: _____

Date: _____

	Satisfactory	Unsatisfactory
1. Carries out Standard Steps A, B, C, D, and E as indicated.	❏	❏
2. Sets up water-seal drainage system.	❏	❏
3. Verifies proper function of water-seal system.	❏	❏
4. Maintains chest tube patency by milking as ordered.	❏	❏
5. Positions system appropriately.	❏	❏
6. Assists patient to turn, cough and deep breathe at least every 2 hours.	❏	❏
7. Marks and records drainage for shift.	❏	❏
8. Assesses function of system frequently.	❏	❏
9. Medicates for pain as needed.	❏	❏
10. Assists with chest tube removal.	❏	❏
11. Applies an air-occlusive dressing to insertion site after tube removal.	❏	❏
12. Carries out Standard Steps X, Y, and Z.	❏	❏

Pass   _____

Fail   _____

Comments: _____

_____

Instructor: _____

© 1994 W.B. Saunders Company. *Rambo's Nursing Skills for Clinical Practice,* fourth edition
All rights reserved.

PERFORMANCE CHECKLIST

Skill 38-10   Assisting with the use of nebulizers

Student: _____

Date: _____

	Satisfactory	Unsatisfactory
1. Carries out Standard Steps A, B, C, D, and E as indicated.	❏	❏
2. Have patient deep breath and cough before beginning treatment.	❏	❏
3. Auscultate lungs.	❏	❏
4. Assist patient to correctly use nasal or oral spray.	❏	❏
5. Set up ultrasonic nebulizer if ordered.	❏	❏
6. Check mist flow, sit patient upright and begin treatment.	❏	❏
7. Monitor patient during treatment.	❏	❏
8. Carries out Standard Steps X, Y, and Z.	❏	❏

Pass _____

Fail _____

Comments: _____

_____

Instructor: _____

© 1994 W.B. Saunders Company. *Rambo's Nursing Skills for Clinical Practice,* fourth edition
All rights reserved.

Suggested Clinical Activities

1. Teach a patient to turn, cough and deep breathe properly to prevent hypoxia.

2. Assist a patient to use an incentive spirometer device.

3. Assist a patient or family member to assume positions for postural drainage of the lungs.

4. Seek assignment to a patient on a ventilator in the clinical setting. Read articles from the suggested reading list to gain more familiarity with ventilators.

5. Observe the various oxygen delivery systems in use on your assigned unit. Ask the patient how he feels about the delivery system.

6. Observe other nurse performing tracheostomy or endotracheal suctioning. Practice this technique in the skill lab if possible.

7. When proficient in endotracheal suctioning, seek opportunities to perform this skill in the clinical setting.

© 1994 W.B. Saunders Company. *Rambo's Nursing Skills for Clinical Practice,* fourth edition
All rights reserved.

Chapter 39

Cardiac Care

LEARNING ACTIVITIES

I. Identify the item in Column I with the label in Column II.

Column I	Column II
_____ 1. P-R interval of .08 sec.	a. normal
_____ 2. heart rate of 48 bpm	b. abnormal
_____ 3. irregular pulse	c. bradycardia
_____ 4. QRS of .20 sec.	d. tachycardia
_____ 5. no visible P wave	e. dysrhythmia
_____ 6. QRS of .08 sec.	
_____ 7. P-R interval of .16 sec.	
_____ 8. heart rate of 126 bpm	
_____ 9. pulse of 88 and regular	
_____ 10. QRS of .04 sec.	

II. Gather some EKG strips from your clinical facility and evaluate them, noting the:

Atrial rate: _____

Ventricular rate: _____

P-R interval: _____

QRS duration: _____

Interpretation: _____

III. Fill in the blank(s) with the correct word(s) or phrase.

1. As depolarization occurs, the cardiac muscle _____.

2. Cardiac monitoring can give information about the following conditions:

   a. _____

   b. _____

   c. _____

   d. _____

   e. _____

© 1994 W.B. Saunders Company. *Rambo's Nursing Skills for Clinical Practice,* fourth edition   625
All rights reserved.

3. Normal electrical conduction in the heart occurs when an impulse arises in the _____.

4. Following conduction the heart has a _____ or _____ period.

5. Depolarization is the _____.

6. A P-R interval is measured from the _____ to the _____.

7. The P-R interval duration is normally _____.

8. Changes in the P-R interval indicate problems in conduction such as _____.

9. Normal QRS duration is _____.

10. An easy way to calculating the heart rate is to count the _____ between two consecutive QRS complexes and divide into _____.

11. Cardiac dysrhythmias are a sign of distubance in the _____ of the impulse or of the _____ of the impulse.

12. Ventricular arrhythmias particularly affect _____.

13. Normal cardiac telemetry monitoring requires the use of _____ leads.

14. During ambulatory cardiac monitoring it must be remembered not to _____.

15. An intra-arterial line provides a continuous direct reading for _____.

16. A pulmonary artery catheter provides information about the function of _____.

17. A pulmonary capillary wedge pressure reading is obtained by _____ of the pulmonary artery catheter.

18. All nurses must be able to identify _____ cardiac dysrhythmias.

19. The cardiac dysrhythmia that most commonly precedes cardiac arrest is _____.

20. Along with cardiac monitoring, the nurse must perform a thorough_____.

IV. Take the post-test included at the end of the chapter in the text.

© 1994 W.B. Saunders Company. *Rambo's Nursing Skills for Clinical Practice,* fourth edition
All rights reserved.

PERFORMANCE CHECKLIST

Skill 39-1   Placement of EKG electrodes for telemetry

Student: _____

Date: _____

	Satisfactory	Unsatisfactory
1. Caries out Standard Steps A, B, C, D, and E as need indicates.	❏	❏
2. Identifies correct sites for desired lead.	❏	❏
3. Cleanses the skin at sites for electrode placement; shaves hair if necessary.	❏	❏
4. Applies the electrodes to the correct sites.	❏	❏
5. Connects telemetry unit wires to correct electrodes for desired lead.	❏	❏
6. Secures the telemetry unit to the patient.	❏	❏
7. Turns on the monitor and checks EKG configuration.	❏	❏
8. Runs a rhythm strip and places it in the patient's chart.	❏	❏
9. Carries out Standard Steps X, Y, and Z.	❏	❏

Pass _____

Fail _____

Comments: _____

_____

Instructor: _____

© 1994 W.B. Saunders Company. *Rambo's Nursing Skills for Clinical Practice,* fourth edition
All rights reserved.

Suggested Clinical Activities

1. Observe a nurse attaching a patient to a cardiac telemetry monitor.

2. Memorize the most common leads used for cardiac telemetry monitoring in your clinical facility.

3. Practice interpreting EKG rhythm strips whenever a chance presents itself.

4. Seek assignment to the critical care unit and observe patients who are undergoing hemodynamic monitoring.

© 1994 W.B. Saunders Company. *Rambo's Nursing Skills for Clinical Practice,* fourth edition
All rights reserved.

Chapter 40

Responding to an Emergency Code

LEARNING ACTIVITIES

I. Fill in the blank(s) with the correct word(s) or phrase.

1. Cardiopulmonary arrest is _____.

2. Respiratory arrest leads to cardiac arrest because _____.

3. Biological death occurs within _____ of cardiac arrest.

4. _____ is the most common cause of cardiopulmonary arrest after myocardial infarction.

5. Every year nearly _____ persons in the U. S. suffer cardiovascular-related deaths.

6. Other conditions that may lead to sudden cardiac death are associated with _____

_____.

7. Cigarrette smoking is a known risk factor for sudden _____.

8. People with chronic deficiencies of _____ and _____ are more prone to cardiac dysrhythmias.

9. Capillary refill is normal when color returns to the nailbed within _____.

10. When working with cardiac patients it is a good idea to get into the habit of each time you pass their door, to look at the _____.

11. The proper technique for checking respirations in a patient who is unresponsive is to _____

    _____.

12. The ABCs of CPR stand for _____.

13. Hyperextension of the head and neck by chin lift and head tilt opens the airway by

    _____.

14. To prevent air build-up in the stomach, breaths need to be given _____.

15. The rate of chest compressions in the adult should be _____.

16. Approximately _____ of normal blood flow can be supplied by chest compressions.

17. The best treatment for ventricular fibrillation is _____.

18. Drugs for dysrhythmias and shock are usually located in _____ of the crash cart.

19. A safety factor when using the defibrillator is not to hold both paddles in one hand; this prevents

    _____.

20. Defibrillator paddles should be placed on the chest with one paddle _____ and the
    other paddle _____.

II. Take the post-test located at the end of the chapter in the text.

© 1994 W.B. Saunders Company. *Rambo's Nursing Skills for Clinical Practice,* fourth edition
All rights reserved.

PERFORMANCE CHECKLIST

Skill 40-1   Checking the equipment and supplies on the "crash cart"

Student: _____

Date: _____

	Satisfactory	Unsatisfactory
1. Obtains inventory checklist.	❑	❑
2. Works from top to bottom of the cabinet.	❑	❑
3. Checks for blank Code blue record forms and checklists.	❑	❑
4. Checks defibrillator correctly.	❑	❑
5. Tests the defibrillator.	❑	❑
6. Checks the EKG paper supply.	❑	❑
7. Checks that backboard is available on side of cart.	❑	❑
8. Completes checklist.	❑	❑

Pass _____

Fail _____

Comments: _____

_____

Instructor: _____

© 1994 W.B. Saunders Company. *Rambo's Nursing Skills for Clinical Practice,* fourth edition
All rights reserved.

PERFORMANCE CHECKLIST

Skill 40-2   Initiating a Code

Student: _____

Date: _____

	Satisfactory	Unsatisfactory
1. Ascertains that person is in need of cardio- pulmonary resuscitation.	❏	❏
2. Calls a "Code".	❏	❏
3. Opens airway.	❏	❏
4. Gives rescue breaths correctly.	❏	❏
5. Checks for circulation.	❏	❏
6. If no pulse, begins compressions and continues rescue breathing in proper sequence.	❏	❏
7. Continues CPR until relieved.	❏	❏
8. Becomes team leader and delegates appropriately.	❏	❏
9. Apprises team of history and physical findings.	❏	❏
10. Assists the team as needed.	❏	❏

Pass _____

Fail _____

Comments: _____

_____

Instructor: _____

© 1994 W.B. Saunders Company. *Rambo's Nursing Skills for Clinical Practice,* fourth edition
All rights reserved.